S0-FEP-712

Better than the Birds
Smarter than the Bees

Better than the Birds *Smarter* than the Bees

No-nonsense Answers to Honest Questions about Sex and Growing Up

Helen Jean Burn

ABINGDON PRESS
NASHVILLE 🙵 NEW YORK

BETTER THAN THE BIRDS
SMARTER THAN THE BEES

Copyright © 1969 by Helen Jean Burn

All rights in this book are reserved.
No part of the book may be reproduced in any
manner whatsoever without written permission of
the publishers except brief quotations embodied in
critical articles or reviews. For information address
Abingdon Press, Nashville, Tennessee.

Library of Congress Catalog Card Number: 69-12771

SET UP, PRINTED, AND BOUND BY THE
PARTHENON PRESS, AT NASHVILLE,
TENNESSEE, UNITED STATES OF AMERICA

Foreword

The insects-and-animals approach to sex has prevailed so long that even in jokes and cartoons "the birds and bees" has become synonymous with sex education.

But in point of fact there is so much more to sex education than the act of reproduction. Human sex involves human beings, individuals with feelings, insecurities, doubts, . . . and questions. During the years of adolescence the need to know and to decide is especially crucial.

This book is based on many face-to-face discussions with young people about sex and growing up, and deals openly and informally with questions and problems which *they* are concerned about as they face a world of difficult choices.

There is no attempt here to provide a sex manual as such or to lay down cut-and-dried rules. Rather the aim is to point to facts, hazards, and possibilities the young person must deal with and to emphasize that as a responsible human being he must make the final decisions.

HELEN JEAN BURN

Acknowledgments

The Planned Parenthood Association of Maryland maintains a speakers' bureau—doctors, nurses, psychiatrists, psychologists, social workers, educators, and clergymen—who appear before groups of young people in order to talk with them and answer their questions. Often these sessions follow a carefully designed series plan. The medical discussions usually come first, followed by those with the social workers and the teachers, with the talks by clergymen completing the series. Thus those young people who come back to their classroom or church or community center for successive sessions have ample opportunities to think through their questions, to develop the feeling of freedom they need in order to ask them, and to reinforce what they are learning by hearing it expressed in different ways by different speakers with differing points of view.

As a social worker specializing in the problems of the young—the promiscuous teen-ager, the unwed mother, the child who cannot be cared for by his natural parents—I was a member of this team of speakers. My own contribution to this book, however, is very small. In the

ACKNOWLEDGMENTS

areas of morality, religion, adolescent psychology, and medicine I am profoundly indebted to the other members of the group.

It would be impossible to give specific credit page by page or even to mention every contributor. Nevertheless, I feel impelled to acknowledge several individuals, because this book leans so heavily upon them. Each is skilled in a particular aspect of the material covered, but the magnitude of his or her contribution rests not so much upon a grasp of the subject matter as upon a rare ability to relate to the young—to establish an almost palpable feeling of closeness with an audience of youngsters (based, I suspect, upon a genuine love for them)—and to *tell it like it is*.

I refer to: Mrs. Vivian Washington, Principal of Baltimore's Public School No. 1 (a facility devoted to the needs of the pregnant teen-ager); the Rev. Frederick J. Hanna, in charge of social services at Emmanuel Episcopal Church in Baltimore; Dr. Claude D. Hill, Obstetrician-in-Chief, Provident Hospital, Baltimore; Dr. Matthew Debuskey, Associate Professor of Pediatrics at The Johns Hopkins School of Medicine, and Chief of the Adolescent Clinic at Sinai Hospital in Baltimore; and Dr. Hugh Davis, Assistant Professor of Obstetrics and Gynecology at The Johns Hopkins School of Medicine. I must assume, however, full responsibility for the material which appears here, for I prepared these pages from my own notes on the sessions.

The extensive bibliography which completes the book is the work of Planned Parenthood's tireless staff, except for the list of fiction relating to the sexual problems of the young; that list was prepared by the Young Adult Department of the Enoch Pratt Free Library in Baltimore.

In closing, I want to express my gratitude to Mrs. Annette Lieberman, the wife of a doctor, the mother of three sons, and the Community Director for the Planned Parenthood Association of Maryland. Her foresight, dedication, efficiency, and unstinting labor formed the backbone of the program upon which this book is based. It is my hope that through these pages her work, and that of the other members of her speakers' bureau, may continue to bear fruit.

Contents

"Doctor—" 11

The Psychological Angle 39

The Boys and the Girls 50

The Marriage Bit 62

Briarpatch Children 71

You and the No-No's 93

Bibliography: Books and Films About Sex 107

"Doctor—"

"Doctor, why didn't the film on reproduction* show anything about people's feelings? I mean, it made it all seem so biological."

Well, you are absolutely right. The film showed sperm wiggling around and eggs and whatnot, and of course to talk about sex in that way only is like looking at the motor of a car instead of considering the trip you are taking. A trip to California is not a lot of pistons going up and down, is it? It involves planning. It involves picking out the right highway. It involves not getting stuck in the mud. It involves having enough money along so that you won't run out of gas. It involves picking very carefully the person who will take the trip with you and being sure that you really want to go on the trip at that particular time.

Certainly all these are things that you want to think

---

* This question-and-answer period was preceded by the showing of a film.

very carefully about. Nevertheless, some understanding of your car's engine will be very helpful to you, and that is why the wise driver wants to learn something about pistons. He has to find out what is normal in the operation of his car so that he can recognize trouble when it occurs. He probably has no intention of making the repairs himself because, if he doesn't know what he is doing, it would be very unwise for him to try. Knowing enough to be able to recognize trouble, however, will alert him to the need to get skilled help when the problems arise.

The same things are true for human reproduction. You are right when you imply there's a very great deal more to this question than biology. An understanding of the biology involved gives you a good foundation for the other areas you must think about—for planning your trip to California wisely. It also will help you to become familiar with what is normal so that when anything abnormal arises, you can get skilled help.

You know, it's a very strange thing, that idea of getting skilled help in regard to the reproductive system. If we have a runny nose and a headache and a fever, we're not reluctant to see a doctor about it. Or, if we get a broken bone or a severe stomach pain, we're not bashful about getting it taken care of. Why should we feel that the reproductive system is so different from the respiratory system or the skeletal system or the gastro-intestinal tract?

There are perfectly good medical names for all the parts and functions of the reproductive system, yet we invent nicknames for these parts and, if we have a question about them, we ask our friends instead of someone who really knows. Films on reproduction should counteract this aura of uncertainty, this feeling of shame and embarrassment. They should help us to look at our bodies in a more natural and wholesome way, and this is a very good thing. Now do any of you have questions about the reproductive system or about the phenomena of intercourse, pregnancy, and birth?

"I'd like to know what causes a miscarriage."

A miscarriage is a loss of the pregnancy prior to what we call "full term." In other words, prior even to a premature birth. The infant is not fully formed and cannot survive. About 10 percent of all pregnancies, for one reason or another, miscarry. In the course of the joining of the sperm and the egg and the implanting of the egg in the wall of the uterus there are many abnormalities that can develop. The really remarkable thing is that it ever works at all—that one tiny fertilized egg can become a whole human being. So it should not be surprising that one out of every ten times something goes wrong. When this happens, nature simply casts off the pregnancy and tries again with a new egg in the next menstrual cycle.

"Is it true that horseback riding or strenuous swimming will make this happen?"

No. Nor will taking hot baths or skipping rope. These are all old wives' tales. There is an arrangement inside the uterus for protecting and cushioning the fetus, a perfectly controlled environment better than any space capsule we've ever been able to design for our astronauts.

"How do people cause abortions?"

You mean illegal abortionists? They reach up inside the uterus and poke around, trying to scrape out the pregnancy. I don't want to frighten you, but these are things you ought to know for your own safety and that of your friends. The illegal abortionist may use a rusty coat hanger or a knitting needle or anything else he has handy. He may poke a hole in the uterus. He may cause a hemorrhage, or a severe infection, or both. Hundreds of women and girls die every year because of this. Just the other day the body of a nineteen-year-old girl was found in the woods over the state line. She had had a criminal abortion which killed her. The person who did it apparently dumped her body there to keep from facing a manslaughter charge, or worse.

In order to protect himself the criminal abortionist will tell the patient that she may feel very sick for a while, but the sick feeling will go away, and she must not tell anyone about it or she will be arrested. The fact is, the person in danger of arrest is the abortionist, and he knows it. Consequently, the patient who suffers these severe after-effects doesn't seek medical help until it's too late. Even those who survive this kind of thing—who manage to get over the infection, the illness, and the pain—often find in later life that their reproductive systems have been so badly damaged they are unable to have children when they want them.

"Aren't some abortions done by regular doctors?"

Yes. It can be done by a doctor when the pregnant woman has, for example, a serious heart ailment that

"DOCTOR—"

might endanger her life or a mental problem which indicates that childbirth at this time would be bad for her. An abortion is a comparatively safe operation, but you understand it must be performed by a skilled doctor in an operating room with the proper equipment and safeguards against infection.

"My girl friend's period never came, and she got a shot and she wasn't pregnant any more. What was that?"

Sterile water, probably. My guess is, she wasn't pregnant at all, just scared. Her period came because the injection relieved her anxiety and tension. There is no shot that can end a pregnancy.

"How do you know when you are pregnant?"

As you saw in the film, when an egg is implanted in the uterus, the menstrual cycle stops. This usually is the first sign—a missed menstrual period. Also, a feeling of nausea, commonly called "morning sickness," may be an early sign that the secretion of hormones in the system has undergone a change. Then, too, the breasts tend to swell and feel different.

"Is that the only reason periods stop?"

No. There are many reasons why a menstrual period may not appear—various irregularities in the way the ovary is functioning. It is wise to get a checkup to establish the cause when this happens.

"Can a girl who hasn't started her periods get pregnant"

It is possible. You see, the menstrual period, or the

15

passing away of the waste material when an egg is not fertilized, is only one phase of the whole menstrual cycle. The egg comes from the ovary and travels down the tube first. In other words, the first egg precedes the first menstrual period or flow. So if a girl is close to the age when her periods are going to begin, she will not know when that first egg appears in the uterus, and she could conceivably become pregnant before her first menstrual flow.

"My gym teacher said you can get pregnant and still be a virgin. Is that true?"

Yes, it is. Obstetricians occasionally see this. A colleague of mine came across three such cases in one month recently. You are all looking horrified. I am not kidding you. It is perfectly possible.

Remember the pictures of the sperm? It has a tail, and it wiggles in what is almost a swimming motion. It actually travels. Now, in every cc.—do you know what a cc. is? It is a cubic centimeter, a little more than half a cubic inch. All right, in every cc. of the fluid discharged from the male during sexual activity there are *100 million* sperm. It takes only one to fertilize an egg.

Now during heavy petting the release of this fluid, or even a little leakage of it prior to the full ejaculation, can take place outside the entrance to the vagina. The sperm can conceivably find its way into the vagina without the male organ actually having penetrated the female, and a girl who has remained technically a virgin can become pregnant.

I assume you all know what I mean by "heavy petting."

"DOCTOR—"

You probably call it something else now, but that's what we used to call it anyway.

"I'm not sure I understand what being a virgin means."

Then you are supposed to ask. The answer takes us back to the film again. You remember, in the pictures of the female anatomy, there was a small membrane covering the opening to the vagina; it is called the *hymen*. Theoretically—at least this is what people believed in the old days—the hymen would remain intact until the female's first experience of sexual intercourse. Actually, with the more athletic life girls live today the stretching or rupture of the hymen comes about naturally, for many girls, before marriage. A century or so ago, however, if a man married a girl and found that the hymen was not intact, he could claim she was not a virgin and call the whole thing off. Now our definition of virginity is a lot more flexible. For us it simply means that the vagina has never been penetrated by the male organ.

"Why do people say that alcohol contributes to sexual promiscuity?"

There is a part of the brain we call the *forebrain*. Animals don't have it; this is why a chimpanzee's head slopes backward. Anyway, you might call this the "don't department of the brain. It tells you, "Don't drive too fast because you may have an accident. Don't throw matches into a can of gasoline or it may explode."

Alcohol affects the brain, and the very first part of the brain it affects is the forebrain, or "don't" department. This results in impaired judgment. You find it increasingly difficult to reason about the consequences of your behavior. Isn't it easy to see then why individuals under the influence of alcohol might do things they would never do under ordinary circumstances?

"We've heard about so many different kinds of birth control. Which do you think is the best method?"

That's easy. Don't have sexual intercourse. Even the safest birth control methods must be used with care, with planning and forethought—with the full use of that "don't" department of the brain. The birth control pills, for example, must be taken faithfully, under a doctor's supervision, for twenty days of the month. If you forget to take them, if you get mixed up about the days, you can get pregnant. Most young people just aren't prepared to do this kind of careful planning. There are psychological factors involved. Some young girls will tell you that while they can imagine being "carried away" on the spur of the moment by a romantic passion, they would feel very uncomfortable about planning ahead for such a moment. That applies also to the other birth control methods, too. What girl, when she meets a really terrific guy at a party, is going to reach into her purse and pull out a diaphragm? And what boy wouldn't be completely turned off by such a sight? That is why I say that until you are mature enough to plan your life wisely, the safest thing to do is keep out of situations which will lead to pregnancy.

"Isn't there supposed to be one pill you can take and be safe?"

"DOCTOR—"

Not yet, and if any of your friends tell you there is, you had better straighten them out about it, too. We are always working on better methods. Maybe someday there will be a single pill or injection or something. But you can be sure that when that time comes, such a method will not be available at the corner drugstore; you will have to get it from a doctor or with a prescription. And this is the way it should be. Medications of that sort are very powerful. They alter the body's customary processes. Years of careful testing must precede their widespread use, and close medical supervision must accompany such use. Doctors want to be extremely careful when they set about altering such a marvelous and mysterious process as the body's reproductive activity.

"People in olden times didn't have anything, did they? I mean, they just had to keep on having children until they were all worn out, didn't they?"

They didn't have what we have. You are right about that. But the use of devices and contraceptive substances was known among ancient tribes and cultures, though these seem to have been far from effective. For many generations knowledge remained on the level prevailing among the Egyptians, Greeks, and Romans. Only in comparatively recent times have scientific means of preventing conception been devised, and the exact time of ovulation been discovered.

"We always hear jokes about 'queers'—you know, homosexuals. Could you tell us about that?"

It means simply that there are some men who are

attracted to other men rather than to the opposite sex, and there are some women who find other women appealing. The causes are not well understood, but they appear to be psychological and to stem from childhood experiences. Many of them can be helped by psychiatric treatment.

You shouldn't joke about them, any more than you ought to joke about any kind of handicap. It is a grave handicap, you know. Because of the very nature of things —the physiology—they are denied normal sexual activity. They do not enjoy the sort of family life the rest of us can look forward to. If their homosexual behavior becomes known, they may be unable to get certain kinds of jobs, or they may lose the jobs they have. They are liable to be arrested, too. It is not a laughing matter.

"Could it happen to any of us?"

You shouldn't worry about it, if that's what you mean. I'm sure many of you girls, when you were young, had mild crushes on other girls or had female teachers you admired. Boys too, in early adolescence often form very strong attachments with other boys. This is usually quite natural.

But with most of us, when we reach a certain age, the proper hormones get turned on, and we discover the opposite sex. The boys become men, and the girls become women, and the whole thing gets straightened out. If, however, you are worried about yourself, get help. Psychological problems seldom go away by themselves—not real problems. If you don't know a psychiatrist or a psychologist to talk to, ask your doctor. It's just like anything else, from pneumonia to transmission trouble in your car, the sooner you get to it, the easier it is to treat.

"Is there really such a thing as an amorph—I can't say the word I mean."

Hermaphrodite. The name comes from Greek mythology. According to the story, Hermes and Aphrodite had a son. When he bathed in a certain fountain, the nymph who lived in the fountain became so enamored of him that she entreated the gods to let her be forever united with him. The result was the formation of a creature who was half-man and half-woman. We use the term hermaphrodite to denote an individual with certain malformations of the sex organs. The condition is extremely rare.

"Can't people have their sex changed now?"

Yes. It sounds very exciting the way they report it in the newspapers. The fact is, it costs a great deal of money, and there are no guarantees. I wouldn't recommend it. It doesn't turn out very well.

What is meant by 'artificial insemination'?"

About 10 percent of the couples who want to have babies find that they cannot, for one reason or another. A gynecologist can work with them. It may simply be a case of the man not having enough sperm at one time, so the doctor can collect it and inject it into the woman at the proper time for her to conceive. In other cases, perhaps as a result of an injury, the man may not be able to provide any sperm at all. It is possible for the doctor to obtain sperm from an anonymous donor and inject it

BETTER THAN THE BIRDS—SMARTER THAN THE BEES

into the woman so that the couple can have a baby.

Unfortunately, legal problems sometimes arise later. Is this baby her husband's child or not? Can the child inherit the husband's money? The courts will probably find ways of straightening these questions out one of these days. In the meantime, gynecologists are giving this sort of help to carefully selected and responsible couples who want it.

"Why didn't the film on reproduction tell about the things that can go wrong, like the diseases you can get?"

I suppose because venereal disease is another subject entirely. But let's talk about it now. Do you all know what we mean by venereal disease? These are diseases transmitted through sexual intercourse, and the two major venereal diseases are gonorrhea and syphilis.

"Where do they come from?"

Do you mean how did the organisms that cause them originate? We don't know. We don't even know where tuberculosis came from, except that you can dig up Egyptian mummies and find evidence that they had it. Is that what you mean?

"No, I heard that syphilis came to this country when the soldiers came back from World War I."

No. It goes back a lot farther than that. Columbus' sailors picked it up from the natives in the New World and carried it to Europe. It had never been known there before, there was no immunity to it or understanding of it, and it spread like wildfire. The French called it the "Spanish disease," and the Spanish called it the "Italian disease," and the Italians called it the "Portuguese disease," and everybody blamed everybody else. It got to be very, very bad. Do you remember seeing in pictures the ladies of the French court wearing beauty marks—little black patches—on their faces? They were using them to cover their syphilis sores. So you see, VD goes back quite a long way.

"Aren't there other ways you can get it, like using dirty rest rooms?"

No. Nor from touching doorknobs. All that is more old wives' tales. I still think it's a good idea to wash your hands often. But you needn't be afraid that everything you touch is going to give you VD.

"Can you get it from kissing people?"

It depends on whom you are kissing. You are certainly not going to get it from kissing your mother. But that brings up another one of the very curious things about human nature. People drop a fork on the floor, and they won't eat with it; but then they'll go out and *kiss* practically anybody. They set up booths at county fairs and start kissing people. I don't know; I just never figured kissing was worth a dollar, considering all the things you might get doing it. Chances are that the floor you dropped the fork on was a lot cleaner than most people's mouths.

There's nothing wrong with kissing, mind you, but I think you ought to be very particular about whom you are kissing, that's all I'm saying. Because, yes, if the person you kiss has a sore in his mouth—a syphilitic sore like the ladies of the French court were hiding with their beauty patches—you can catch the disease from that person without going any further than kissing them.

"Can a fellow tell if the girl he's going with has VD?"

No, he can't, unless he sees a sore and can recognize what it is—which he probably can not do. You certainly mustn't go around accusing people with skin blemishes of having VD. Only a medical examination, including laboratory tests, can make the diagnosis. The best test for the boy to make is to ask himself honestly what kind of a girl she is. Is she likely to have been going with a lot of other fellows, who in turn have been running around with a lot of other girls, and so on? VD thrives in an atmosphere of promiscuity. The people who get it tend to live this kind of life. They do not generally have any serious attachments to their sex partners; they just go from one to the other.

It's rather like a person with a very bad cold. If he goes down the row and coughs in your face, and then in your neighbor's face, and then in the next one's face, pretty soon he can fix the whole room up with a bad cold.

"That means then—I'm still thinking about the kissing part—that wearing a male contraceptive, a rubber, will not protect you from getting a disease, doesn't it?"

Well, it won't *hurt*. When the fellow with the cold coughs in your face, it certainly will help if you turn away, or if he covers his mouth. It seems sensible to expose yourself as little as possible. But of course the safest thing of all is to keep away from the problem entirely. Failing that, if you are going to run with that sort of people, you most assuredly should do the best you can to protect yourself. For the male that sort of contraceptive will certainly help.

"DOCTOR—"

"Could a person be a carrier of VD and not actually have it?"

No. You can't give it to somebody unless you've got it, but it is possible for a girl to have gonorrhea or syphilis and not know it. If a boy has gonorrhea, he can't miss it. But syphilis is a rather subtle disease. It works silently. The classic first symptom is a small sore. It isn't particularly painful. You may not even notice it. In a girl it may appear inside the vagina where she almost certainly would not detect it. After a while the sore goes away, and if you were aware of it at all, you would believe your troubles were over.

Actually, the spirochete—the bacteria which causes syphilis—is in the bloodstream. It travels in somewhat the same way the sperm does. It sort of undulates through the bloodstream and works its way into the various vital organs. The only way to find out it is there is with a blood test. Meanwhile, the individual who does not know he or she has it could have been infecting dozens of others with it.

"You say that with gonorrhea, you know you've got it. How do you know?"

First of all, by learning enough about your own body to know what is normal. It is not normal to have a discharge —a leakage of fluid—from the penis of the male. If you find that your underclothing is being soiled by a yellowish discharge, you know that is not normal and should be looked into. In the female at certain times in the menstrual cycle there may be a small amount of white discharge, and this is normal. But any change in this, an increase or a difference in the color, ought to be investigated medically.

Not every discharge, of course, is venereal disease. But only competent medical attention will be able to ascertain whether the discharge you are having is actually VD or something else.

In addition, gonorrhea causes painful complications in the male. A person suffering from it has to get up frequently in the night to urinate, and it burns and is very painful, so he is usually willing to go to the doctor about it.

"If you go to the doctor and he finds you have VD, must you tell him where you got it?"

You should, as—to use the term you hear on television all the time—a public service.

The only way to stop this problem is to catch up with everyone who has it and treat them. Perhaps it would help if you thought of it in terms of the golden rule. If you had syphilis, if those spirochetes were wiggling around in your bloodstream, wouldn't you want to know? You see, that is the part only you can do; getting yourself, and everyone else who needs it, in for treatment. Penicillin, while not foolproof, does a job on VD. But the number of cases is increasing anyway. In our own city it has increased *200 percent* in the last six years among people under the age of nineteen.

All the penicillin in the world won't help if the individuals who have the diseases don't come in and get it. And believe me, venereal disease will not go away all by itself. It has got to be treated.

"DOCTOR—"

"Once you get one of these diseases and penicillin cures it, are you immune from then on?"

No, you are not. It isn't like chicken pox. You can go out and get it again the next week, and get that cleared up, and go out again the next week, and so on. Only there's a limit to how much penicillin some patients can take. This is something the doctor must manage with care. He knows that a time may come when you have pneumonia and really need penicillin to save your life. He doesn't want you to have reached a point where he can't give it to you then.

"How long does it take to get rid of VD?"

That depends first on how long you've had it before you get it attended to. Just as an example, let's suppose you find the first symptom on a Monday morning, and you go to see a doctor on Monday night. If he is in an office or clinic where laboratory service is available on the spot, he might have his diagnosis complete that same evening and begin treating you at once. Within forty-eight hours the disease could be under control. Of course, in order to prove that it is further tests would be necessary later on. Very prompt early treatment of both gonorrhea and syphilis definitely cut down on the time you need to spend in clearing up the trouble.

"If that's all there is to it, why do our teachers keep telling us VD is so horrible?"

The question we doctors keep asking ourselves is, if that's all there is to it, why don't people who have been exposed to VD come in and get themselves treated?

27

Because, you see, they don't. That's what makes VD so "horrible," as you say.

Let's consider gonorrhea first. When gonorrhea goes untreated, it spreads through the urinary and the reproductive systems. I've told you about the discomfort. In addition there may be fever. It is a full-scale infection. In the female this infection spreads up into the uterus and into the Fallopian tubes, which carry the eggs from the ovaries to the uterus. In these tubes the infection causes a pocket of pus—a boil, in effect. The tube swells. There is a good deal of pain and fever and discharge. But worse than that, if this inflammation isn't treated right away, the tube tends to become scarred and damaged so that it cannot transport the eggs later on. There is a good chance that a woman who has suffered such an infection will be unable to have children when she wants them.

The long-range effects of syphilis, however, are far worse. I wish I had some pictures to show you, because this is one of those times when one picture is definitely worth a thousand words. Here again I have no wish to give you nightmares, but these are things you need to know.

When those spirochetes I described to you go traveling through the bloodstream, they get into the spinal column, the heart, the liver, the brain. They just go all over, and this becomes a chornic affair that goes on for years and years and years. It has been the cause of very serious trouble in the vital organs and in the central nervous system, sometimes resulting in paralysis and even insanity, to say nothing of shortening the patient's life in addition to incapacitating him.

"DOCTOR—"

Under normal circumstances you young people can expect to live very long, healthy lives—longer and healthier than those of my generation. What the promiscuous teenager is messing around with is his or her future. You have plenty of time to make sensible decisions about your life and your health. Just because everything seems to be speeded up and pushed ahead these days—things like drinking and driving—does not mean you've got to cram everything in at once. Think about the eighty years or so of your life as a whole, and take time to use your head.

Now you are thinking, here comes the sermon. All right, I'll quit preaching about preserving your life. What you do with it is your own business. But believe me when I say that syphilitic brain damage is no way to go.

"Is this another one of those old wives' tales, or is it true that if a pregnant woman has syphilis, her baby can be born with it?"

That is true, and very tragic. It results in deformed bodies, blindness, mental retardation, skin disease. Fortunately, we don't see nearly as much of this as we used to, because now blood tests are made on pregnant women. That gives the doctor a chance to get to work on the problem fairly early in the pregnancy. However, if a pregnant girl does not seek medical attention because she is afraid of letting her condition become known, then the problem could go undetected until it is too late to prevent malformation of the baby, or whatever form the disease—which, incidentally, is called congenital syphilis—happened to take.

"Is that why in a lot of states you can't get a marriage license without a blood test?"

That's right. It is simply a safeguard for both partners in the marriage and for the children they may have.

Young lady in the second row, you look puzzled. Have I confused you in some way?

"No, I was just thinking that this is the kind of thing that can come from having intercourse—I mean, it makes you think maybe it would be better not to get married, or anything, at all."

I *have* confused you, I see. Let me say this very clearly: venereal disease is not caused by sexual intercourse itself, but by *promiscuity*. Just because there is an occasional rotten apple in the market, you don't give up eating apples. You can take a whole barrel of apples and not find a single rotten one. On the other hand, you can put one rotten apple in a barrel, and it can spoil the whole containerful, especially if the apples inside the barrel are being stirred around and knocked against each other all the time, if you get my message.

Suppose you are going with a crowd of people. All it takes is for one of them to take a trip down to the red-light district of the town, and this one individual can come back and give VD to a couple of people in the crowd. They give it to four more of their friends, who in turn give it to eight others, and so on. This sort of activity is what we mean by promiscuity. There is rarely any love in it; there are no lasting attachments—do you see what I mean? Nobody in that crowd, to go back to my earlier illustration, is planning his trip to California

"DOCTOR—"

with any kind of forethought or care. They are engaging in sexual intercourse for no reason other than the ready availability of the opposite sex.

This has nothing whatever to do with mature, self-controlled people who genuinely love each other, who want to plan their lives together, who want to enjoy the tenderness and beauty of sexual relations which are an outgrowth of true affection and unselfish consideration. For them, going to bed together is only one aspect of a larger relationship involving the entire personalities of both. They derive as much joy from being kind to one another, from taking long walks together, from sharing their inmost thoughts and feelings, as they do from physical intimacy. This is what we mean by real love, and it is surely the greatest joy to be found anywhere in the whole range of human experience.

Compared to this, promiscuous sex is as phony and as valueless as a three-dollar bill. It shouldn't even go by the same name. Don't make the mistake of confusing the two kinds of sex in your thoughts. And don't let fear deprive you of the right kind of sexual relationship when the proper time for it comes in your life. Above all, don't let the heedlessness of these hurrying teen-age years get you into the sort of trouble that could spoil your chances of attaining enduring joy later on.

"Can we go back to talking about pregnancy for a minute? I read in the paper that in our city every week twenty-five girls have to drop out of school because they are going to be unwed mothers. Is this because teen-agers are getting awfully wild all of a sudden?"

I don't think that's all there is to it. Some experts say things are no different now, only we aren't hiding them anymore. Personally, I believe this is only half true. We are talking more about sex. We are feeling less embarrassed about these things. Certainly there are some very explicit movies and magazines available now. I think more young people are experimenting now than ever before. The reason may be that while the rather irresponsible elements in our culture (publishers of pornography, for example) are going wild with their wares, the rest of us haven't moved fast enough in educating young people about themselves.

But there is another element in this, too. Medical studies have shown that girls are reaching childbearing age somewhat earlier than they used to. For example, a hundred years ago the average age for the start of the first menstrual period was approximately fifteen. Now it's around thirteen-and-a-half. This may be the result of our better nutrition and our better general health—although there is some doubt there too, because it has been found that in countries where there is not enough nutritious food, the birth-rate does not go down.

It would appear that nature is determined to propagate the human race, whether there is enough food to go around or not. The reproductive system will rob the rest of the body in order to keep itself functioning. Calcium, for example, will be used to make the baby grow while the mother's teeth decay. So we are a long way from getting all the answers we need in this area.

Nevertheless, good general health certainly does not make you less fertile, that's for sure. Perhaps it is safe to

"DOCTOR—"

assume that a longer childbearing period is related to our modern vitamins and the prevention of disease through vaccination. Whatever the reason, it is a fact that nature seems to be trying to get you pregnant. Remember, in the female a new egg is produced each and every month from the time the girl is about thirteen until she gets into her middle or late forties. And remember also those 100 million sperm in every cc. of the male's seminal fluid. In view of this, it is not surprising that young people who engage in sexual intercourse have an excellent chance of producing babies. Some girls who have gotten pregnant will tell you "it only happened once," and you probably will not believe them. But it is entirely possible, just as we have pointed out that it is possible for a girl to become pregnant without ever having experienced the complete sexual act.

"Then why is it we all know girls who are really, really pigs, and yet they never get pregnant?"

Maybe they know more about birth control than you do. Or maybe their tubes have already been damaged by venereal disease.

"Well, if young girls are so healthy now, why do they talk about 'risk' pregnancy?"

High-risk pregnancy. That's the term we use. It's because no matter how healthy she may be, a teen-ager is not fully grown. Her bone structure isn't fully formed. I told you the reproductive system will rob the mother's body of nutritional elements. This means that a very young girl who is pregnant needs more than ever to eat properly.

33

Soft drinks and potato chips won't supply what she needs.

There are a number of medical problems we must pay attention to in this type of pregnancy, and so often the girl who is unmarried is the one who will not go to a doctor or a clinic promptly because she doesn't want her condition known. The sad thing is that she, of all pregnant women, most needs early and close medical supervision.

"You hear jokes about this, and I wish you'd explain about it: Why does it hurt a fellow to stop after he's gotten hot?"

That's true, there is some discomfort, and it's no joke. You see, there are two main blood vessels in the penis. One is the artery that brings the blood in, and the other is the vein that takes it out. When the boy becomes sexually aroused, hormones are secreted which cause the vein to close off. The blood in the penis builds up. This makes possible the stiffening of the organ that we call erection and enables the penetration of the female's vagina. If the sex act is not completed, this buildup of blood becomes somewhat uncomfortable. It is a feeling of fullness or pressure which ebbs away slowly.

"Is there anything you can do about it?"

You might think about something else and do calisthenics. This is where the jokes come in about boys going down the street lifting up car bumpers. The idea is to get unexcited by putting your mind on something else and to increase the general circulation of the blood.

Better than such a method, though, is not to let your

"DOCTOR—"

making-out (or whatever you kids are calling it this year) go that far. And this brings us to something we haven't done much talking about. I mean the need for a better understanding—and hence a better management—of your own sex drive.

What I am talking about now applies mainly to the boys, but much of it needs to be understood by the girls as well.

In your early life the male penis serves mainly as an excretory organ which passes urine from the body. As you reach young adulthood, or puberty, it begins to serve a two-fold purpose; passing urine and reproduction. As a part of the second function certain hormones begin to be produced in the body which bring about some rather radical changes. For example, when the male testicles begin to produce the male hormones, we find that our stature and muscular development increase markedly. The voice deepens. We begin to grow hair over the body and on the face. Eventually we have to begin to shave.

In addition to these physical changes that we can see, there are certain psychological changes also. They are definitely related to the emergence of the male hormone in the system, and one of these effects is the appearance of sexual desire. This sexual stimulation should be looked at in a broad sense. It is more than the mechanism of erection and intercourse.

Let's use the word *push*. This emerging maleness begins to give us the push that makes us want to work hard, to be constructive and creative. It makes us want to become successful wage-earners and eventually leads us into marriage and the production of children in this marriage.

BETTER THAN THE BIRDS—SMARTER THAN THE BEES

All of this is a part of the sex drive. It is not limited to the performance of a simple sex act but includes the whole pattern of our lives as men.

You see, we are not birds and bees, and it is extremely short-sighted of us to talk about the human sex drive in terms of the birds and the bees. Any animal, no matter how low on the scale of intelligence, can perform the sex act. You can take a frog and sever the connection between the brain and the spinal cord, and still that frog can engage in reproduction. It doesn't take a brain or any intelligence at all to have intercourse.

What does require intelligence is controlling the sex drive and using it wisely. This wealth of *push* that derives from the phenomena of emerging sexuality in humans can be channeled into constructive activity. It can be used. It will not be depleted, but it can be used in other ways. Some of these other ways are found in athletic endeavors. Participating in strenuous physical activities which involve competition with other boys or with yourself, in bettering your own performance, is an excellent way of putting this great push you have to use. Working hard at your studies, doing science projects, and working on the school newspaper—all of these activities serve as constructive uses for your emerging drives. So do hobbies, school committees and clubs, and normal, wholesome recreational pursuits like dances, picnics, hikes, and parties.

You must remember that you are not a frog, driven by blind, purely animal urges. You are a whole human being, and your sex drive is an integral part of your entire personality. A teenager who is interested in nothing but

"DOCTOR—"

sex is more of an animal than a human being. And the few individuals of that type who exist are not at all well.

"What causes 'wet dreams'?"

The seminal fluid builds up, and this is nature's way of releasing it. It is perfectly natural. Usually, and possibly always, it is accompanied by a dream involving sexual activity. You may forget the dream when you wake up, but there will be a stain on your clothing to indicate that the discharge of the fluid from the penis has taken place. The whole thing is as natural and normal as the menstrual period or going to the bathroom.

This may be a good place to discuss masturbation, too. Most all children when they are small discover their own genitals and are curious about them. In the old days people used to believe this was very naughty. If they found their son or daughter touching his or her organs, punishment would follow. This made the child feel very guilty, and often these guilt feelings gave him problems in regard to his own sexuality later in life.

Now we are more enlightened about this. Curiosity and even manipulation of your own sex organs will not drive you insane; it will not make you incapable of normal sexual activity in the future; and it does not mean you are abnormal or dirty in any way. It is just another aspect of emerging sexuality—a very minor aspect, I might add. I have yet to see a study which gave evidence that masturbation ever did any *good*, and I think what I said before about channeling your urges into constructive activities applies here as well. If you are going to spend a lot of time alone in your room, you would do well to collect stamps or get yourself a chemistry set. That way, your spare time will be considerably more educational, and you'll have something tangible to show for it.

I think the time has come to do a little summing up, and if you are not now sick of the subject of frogs, I'd like to talk about them just once more.

Those of you who have had a chance to watch, in a tank in your science class, the phenomenon of gluey-looking little eggs becoming wiggly tadpoles and then turning into complete frogs with fully formed and powerful legs know something of the wonderful changes nature brings about. In this frog cycle the most exciting time is when the slippery little adolescent frogs are trying to stop being tadpoles and breathing like fish and are attempting to climb out of the water onto a rock and be real, jumping, air-breathing frogs. It is a critical time in their lives. A lot of them don't make it. Even for those that do, it isn't easy.

Adolescent humans go through a similar transition. You find your problem not in trying to climb up on a rock, but in learning to accept and live with and manage your own sexuality. Many adults of the human species may have forgotten what a difficult climb this is, but not all have. Many of us want very much to give you a hand up onto that dry, sunny rock. Don't be ashamed to ask for it.

Try to make wise decisions for yourself. Don't let yourself slip into troublesome situations. But if you do slip, by all means yell for help, and yell very, very promptly.

The Psychological Angle

"Isn't it a fact that after you reach a certain age, if you don't have sex, you'll go crazy?"

No, it isn't. Sex is a drive, not an appetite like hunger or thirst. You can control it. You can postpone it. You can abandon it completely without ill effects. You will not die. You will not become psychotic.

As a matter of fact, the major difficulties in this area come from trying to use sex to solve nonsexual problems. So much of today's sexual activity is simply an attempt to find a tranquilizer for anxiety. The individual feels inadequate in his work or in his homelife, so he uses sex to try to make himself feel better. It never works for long.

For some people sex may be the only way they *know* of relating to another person. They may indulge in sex on the first date simply because they have nothing to talk about. The sad thing is that in this sort of relationship there is no real communication. It's like—have you ever seen very small children playing in a room together? Two-year-olds don't really play together; they play side by side, each in a private world. That's the way the sexual activity I'm talking about works. It's really autoeroticism—loving themselves, satisfying themselves—it just happens to take place in the same place and at the same time for two people who actually have no relationship to each other.

"Then what's the answer? What does it take to be able to communicate?"

In the area of sex it takes more than the simple proximity of the appropriate organs. It takes mutual interests and respect and affection and time. I guess the word for all this is "love." Or is that old-fashioned?

"As far as guys are concerned, I don't think sex has anything at all to do with love. I mean you can be interested in a girl for sex when you hardly even like her, and you can like another girl a whole lot and leave her alone."

All right, that is true for the male. But we are talking about communication, about relationships with some kind of meaning, and about not using sex selfishly.

"Well, what's wrong with using sex, if you need it?"

The real question is, what do you need? Is it the physiological mechanism of the sex act, or is it something else? Is it love you need or—if you don't like that word—is it a feeling of being considered important and worthwhile by some other human being? Is it confidence you need? I am saying you can't use sex to solve nonsexual problems. I am saying you should try to figure yourself out so you know what you are really seeking when you spend time

THE PSYCHOLOGICAL ANGLE

with a girl you don't even like. Because to go back to the first question, you don't need sex, not literally, the way you need food and water.

"Aren't there people who do, people like sex maniacs, nympho——"

Nymphomaniacs. Yes, there are abnormal people. The abnormality is not physical or chemical though as far as we can tell. It's psychological, which means they are seeking something else, a love denied them in childhood or revenge on someone who hurt them. The fact that sex is not what they really need is proven by the fact that they never get enough.

"I can't imagine sex without love. Most girls I've talked to feel the same way. Is it really true that boys are completely different? That makes us feel that we can't ever be sure they mean what they say."

You can't deny the vast difference between the male and female attitude toward sex; it would be foolish to try. And when I spoke a moment ago about what it is we are seeking when we seek sex, I didn't mean to oversimplify. Let me go back and clarify some of this.

In the earlier history of man (and even now in what we call primitive societies) there were actual ceremonies and rites involved in growing up. When a boy learned to hunt and fish and fight, he was taken in hand by adult men and initiated with elaborate ceremonies into the status of manhood. Now to achieve adulthood, much more is required. You've got to learn to drive a car. You've got to earn money. You've got to go to school long

41

past the onset of physical puberty. It's no wonder the adolescent boy feels insecure and confused about his status in the tribe. He may be drafted before he can buy a drink or be trusted by his father with the family car. Why should we be shocked if he feels a need to prove his manhood, or if the method he selects for his test is sexual prowess? What he is doing is collecting scalps to hang in his lodge. Hunting girls is easier than hunting buffalo and eagles—and it's more fun! Nevertheless, he is still following an ancient pattern.

The girls are still following an ancient pattern too, and that's where the difference lies. The psychological makeup of the female still reflects the era when her primary function was to preserve the race through bearing and raising young. Now in an age of overpopulation, contraceptives, and careers for women, this may be very much out-of-date; but it is true, nevertheless. A woman looks for security. Fortunately, by the time the male has collected a few scalps and feels surer of his manhood, he begins to look for security, too. The man and woman get married as a result of an eventual agreement as to their aims in life. During their adolescent period though, we should not be surprised if the boy and girl do not see eye to eye.

"Is that why—I'm thinking about the woman wanting security—some girls say they don't get much out of sex?"

That is probably true. That and the emotional effect of the sex act itself. What I mean is, the young man may seem very attentive beforehand while afterwards he is so relaxed and sleepy he doesn't feel like talking. The girl— particularly the unmarried girl who has mixed feelings

THE PSYCHOLOGICAL ANGLE

about sex outside of marriage, who may not be comfortable in the sort of places in which their love-making must take place, and who can never be sure about the genuineness of his feeling for her unless he is willing to marry her —this girl is in great need of reassurance, especially afterward. If she doesn't get it, she will quite understandably feel disheartened, let down. She may be troubled by the feeling that she is cheap. She may feel guilty. She may very well feel that this sex business is simply not what it's cracked up to be.

"I heard somewhere that a girl who gets pregnant when she is not married really wanted a baby anyway. Is that true?

Maybe she did not consciously want a baby, but she wanted something she was not getting. It's still the same subject we were discussing a while ago: she is using sex in an effort to find something else. I won't go into the things we know about the unwed teen-age mother now, but I will say that a great many young, pregnant schoolgirls have similar emotional problems, and, yes, some of them do show a deep need to prove themselves by giving birth to a baby. It's not much different from the manhood-proving we talked about earlier.

"All the kids I know who go in for sex in a big way hate at least one of their parents. What's the connection? I think they are trying to get even."

You may be right. What do the rest of you think? Do parents do things which drive their children into extreme behavior? And, if so, what are some of the things these parents do?

"They keep harping on your appearance, your clothes and your hair."

"They treat you like an infant."

"They call you names all the time, hood, bum, tramp."

"They accuse you and your friends of a whole lot of things you haven't done. They say you are no good—so you figure you might just as well go out and do what they accuse you of."

All right, good. Now think about some of the things we have been saying. Think of some of the motives behind sexual activity, and let's see how they relate to these problems with parents.

"They are saying we aren't grown up enough to belong to the tribe."

"They are making us feel unloved, so we look for love someplace else."

That's right. I can't change the attitudes of your parents; their respect is something you must earn. And I won't kid you, there are parents with severe problems, too. Maybe there are cases where no matter what the kid does he isn't going to be able to change his parents' attitude. But at least you can be honest with yourself. When you go out with somebody you don't even like, don't pretend it is because your sex drive is too strong for you to cope with. Admit you are trying to prove something, or maybe that you long for a friend—one real good friend who understands you.

"Yeah, but aren't you supposed to want to get away from your folks? Isn't that the way things should be?"

Certainly, and a lot of adolescent rebellion is a perfectly healthy attempt to get out of the nest. Ideally, it should be painless. It shouldn't lead you into a lot of extreme behavior like stealing hubcaps or drunken driving or getting pregnant out of wedlock.

"Don't you think teen-agers have sexual relationships for the same reasons that they drink and smoke and take drugs and drive too fast? Don't you think they are trying to seem older and smarter than they really feel?"

Yes. It's a common human fallacy—put on the appearance of something you are not, and maybe you will become that thing. Perhaps a more charitable way of saying it would be: They are attempting to assume an adult male or female role. On some kids it is actually pitiful; they are like little children playing dress-up. It is pitiful because they are simply not prepared to assume responsibility for the consequences of their acts. They begin by trying to punish their parents or establish their independence from their parents, and end by making such a mess of their lives that they become more dependent than ever.

"Personally, I really don't see why the powers that be won't just let young people have contraceptives and go ahead and do what they want. Then everybody would be happy."

The trouble is, it just isn't that simple. First of all, there isn't a perfect contraceptive. Each of the various kinds has advantages and disadvantages, and all of them have to be used with great care. The conflict between "sex" and "love" comes up here. If both people involved frankly are interested in nothing but sex, maybe they can be very cool about the contraceptive question. I heard about one girl who was asked, "What do you say if the guy refuses to wear a rubber?" and she replied, "I tell him to go to hell!" There aren't many teen-aged girls who manage their lives that efficiently.

Consequently, for both the male and the female venereal disease is a hazard. And for the girl pregnancy is a hazard. So contrary to the conclusion you present in your question, unlimited promiscuity does not by any means guarantee that everyone is going to be happy.

"You keep mentioning love, and then we get away from it again. If such a thing as sex based on love is possible, what would be wrong with that, at any age?"

Nothing, if love were easily recognizable. Adolescents are very much interested in love. They can love very deeply for maybe three or four months at a time. The trouble is, a sexual relationship often ends by committing you to much more of a relationship than a happy three- or four-month episode. When things go wrong, you are back where you started, or maybe worse off. The boy has a scalp for his lodge, but often he has a lot of guilt feelings, too. And the girl is more insecure than ever, just because a relationship she believed in didn't last. And perhaps the parents are still saying "hood!" and "tramp!" only now it hurts more than ever.

"Well, I think the sick people are the adults. You don't see teen-agers going to bunny clubs and topless nightclubs and places like that."

THE PSYCHOLOGICAL ANGLE

I'm glad you brought that up. We must never fall into the trap of saying, "Naughty, naughty kids." The fact is, those sexy movies and nude photographs and pornographic magazines are made by adults whose sole aim in life is to make money. In a very real sense they are the sick ones in our society. But every person has to make the ultimate decisions on his own. You ought to have more help than you are getting; that is certainly true. Still, at some point the opportunity to do exactly what you want to do is going to be there. Nothing that we say now will guarantee your choice in advance. You can't be programmed like a computer. All that the people who care about you can hope for is that you will make an intelligent choice, based on some understanding of yourself, of what you really want and what you really need. That's why I keep talking about honesty. If you are honest with yourself, you have a better chance of making choices you can live with.

"I think maybe the big change in our time is our honesty. I don't think we are doing much that is different —we just don't hide what we do. Young people, I mean. We are trying to be honest about our feelings. We are trying to be open and natural about sex. Isn't it psychologically healthier to lie down on the grass in the park and make out, than to sneak up the back stairway to your secretary's apartment after dark?"

All right, let's get something straight. Teen-agers are not the only people with sex problems. The really severe sex problems that wind up in the office of a shrink are often the result of something we hope is dying—bad sex education. This sort of sex education used to be the only kind of sex education anybody ever got: it involved such things as making a child feel like a filthy little animal if he were caught masturbating. As for using sex to prove something, you ought to see the spectacle of a middle-aged man having an extramarital affair to convince himself that age has not weakened his virility.

I could go farther. I might be justified in saying that although teen-agers have a lot of problems, very often sex is not one of them. Certainly sex is not a problem for the young person with the perfectly honest and free attitude you describe. Maybe he is troubled by loneliness; maybe he feels inadequate to deal with his life as a whole; but sex, in itself, is not a problem for him.

The question in my mind is, how many young people like that are there, really? The fact is, the old education has not yet died out completely. We haven't entirely shaken off the guilt. And we may never succeed in shaking off the ancient security-oriented attitude, the one that makes a woman yearn for a safe haven for her mating and that eventually leads a man to want to settle down in that safe haven with her.

The boy who keeps telling himself what a swinger he is may on a deeper level be very unsatisfied with the way he lives. He may be pursuing a series of promiscuous relationships, not because he truly wants to, but because of the pressure put on him by the others in his group. You see, the pendulum has swung all the way among many groups of young people. Whereas a generation ago the social pressure was to live a blameless life on the surface and to conceal any messing around you did, now an individual known to lack sex experience is in the Out Crowd. This kind of motivation is just as phony as the middle-aged boss who sneaks up his secretary's back stairs after dark. What I mean is, his hiding an affair from public opinion is no more false than your putting up a big free-love front so you won't be called a square. Again it is using sex to solve a nonsexual problem.

"It really doesn't seem important to me what older people are doing. I think girls my age feel things more. I think things hurt us in a way that older people don't feel."

Yes, of course. That is why the wrong sort of sex—the loveless, uncommunicative sort of sex—is not what you need. That sort of sex is anything but reassuring. It is anything but beautiful. It can be unglamorous, joyless, desperate; and very, very lonely.

The Boys and the Girls

"Is it up to the boy or the girl to draw the line?"

Like table tennis, the tango, and the seesaw, it takes *two*.

Because a man's physical strength is superior to a woman's, the man's role is appropriately that of a protector. When a boy takes a girl out on a date, he is assuming responsibility for her safety. Even our manners acknowledge this by directing him to open the door for her, walk on the curb side of the pavement, and help her across the street. Although a boy may not observe all these small formalities, he nevertheless would want to be able to defend his date from some hood who made insulting remarks to her or tried to harm her. She would certainly expect this of him, and so would her parents. If he failed her in a crisis, they would have a very low opinion of him, and he would have a very low opinion of himself. Isn't it natural then to expect him to protect her from himself as well? Both kinds of protection require the same sort of strength. We usually call it manhood.

Now what of the girl's part in this? Let's go back to the imaginary situation where a couple of hoods try to take the girl down an alley. Would the girl stand by, blubbering, while her date fought them off alone, or would she try to help in some way? I think most girls would look for a way to help, don't you? Well, when her date's struggle is with himself, he needs help, too.

Not long ago I heard a doctor say that in all the years of a man's life his sexual urge is greatest during his late teens. He has the most powerful sex drive he will ever have at a time when he has the least experience in learning to control it. "Nature," the doctor remarked, "has played a dirty trick on the teen-ager."

It is important that the girl refuse to take part in nature's "dirty trick." Further, she needs to help the boy by drawing the line and holding it.

This requires honesty on her part. She should ask herself just how much of his physical desire she has deliberately tried to arouse. Has she dimmed the lights and turned the music low in the hope that he will ask her to the next school dance? Has she let their movie date end up in some dark parking spot so that he might give her his class ring?

If she has, she's joined the opposition just as surely as if she had started fighting on the side of the hoods in that alley.

"Why do girls wear short skirts and tight sweaters and stand real close to a guy all the time they're talking to him, if they're going to start fighting him off later on? Doesn't it seem like they're saying 'no' at 11 p.m. after saying 'yes' all day?"

It does, but it probably isn't deliberate. After all, Sadie Hawkins' Day comes but once a year. The girl has very little opportunity to ask a boy out. She's got to attract his attention someway, or he may never notice her at all. She's got competition, too. Other girls are trying to get his eye.

Most girls don't go out looking for sex. They are looking for attention, for popularity. They want very much to be liked. They genuinely believe the way to be liked is to dress in the manner you describe. When Miss Miniskirt walks into homeroom, and a guy's eyes light up, she doesn't know it's because his glands have started pumping hormones into his bloodstream. She thinks he *likes* her.

When she cuddles up to him beside his locker, she's trying to make sure he doesn't get a chance to look at anybody else. The remotest thing from her mind is his pulse rate.

Now if his blood pressure were normal and his respiration not quite so labored, he might be able to figure it all out. Boys *do* know how girls are, or they wouldn't whisper sweet nothings to them when they really have their minds on something else. But in his state he isn't thinking very clearly. The message she is transmitting is not the message he is picking up. And when the whole thing culminates in an 11:00 p.m. wrestling match, no one is more surprised than Miss Miniskirt. She simply cannot understand what got into him.

It really boils down to the boy's and girl's mutual ignorance of each other's basic nature.

"Don't some girls use sex as a weapon against boys?"

THE BOYS AND THE GIRLS

Yes, some of them do. They are the barracudas in the sea of sex. They are more merciless than any man-eating shark.

What a girl like that wants is power. She enjoys getting as many boys going for her as she possibly can. Then she treats them mean just for fun. But once her tactics become clear any guy who keeps going back for more is a poor fish indeed.

"Why do boys say one thing in the dark and something else in the daylight? They give a girl a big line about how everybody is doing it, and this is the twentieth century, and there's absolutely nothing wrong with going all the way. But they really don't mean it, because once a girl has given in to them they act like she's just dirt. I know one boy who told his kid sister he'd break her neck if he ever caught her messing around, and yet that same guy goes out every weekend and messes around himself!"

And if anybody should tell him he's being dishonest, he wouldn't believe it, would he?

Let me explain a boy like that to you. He thinks it's all a game and that he is playing by the rules. It doesn't seem immoral to him, any more than an ordinary athletic contest seems immoral. Take lacrosse, for example. It's a series of acts of violence, punctuated by the referees' whistles. This boy we're talking about would never think of running along a crowded street, brandishing a big stick and knocking pedestrians out of his way. He knows that's not acceptable behavior. He does it in lacrosse because that's the way you play the game. A certain amount of brutality is perfectly suitable.

The reason he feels no pangs of conscience about lying to a girl in the back seat is because he doesn't think of boy-girl relationships in the same way that he thinks of an orderly, well-regulated city street where individuals behave with some mutual respect and sense of responsibility. Rather, he thinks of boy-girl relationships as just another body-contact sport. The goal happens to be the girl's surrender. If she is really fond of him, and especially if she is less experienced than he is, that's fine. It makes it all the easier to score.

He is ignoring a fundamental difference though. When the game in the back seat gets too rough, there's nobody around to blow the whistle. And in his heart this boy knows he isn't being fair. When he counseled his sister, he was really saying to her, "Watch out for guys like me. They play dirty."

"Is it true that most fellows, no matter what kind of a line they give you, really want you to say 'no'?"

It might be more accurate to say that within any boy, a part of him wants the girl to say "yes," and a part of him wants her to say "no." What she must decide is which part of his nature she wants to please, which part of his nature she can depend on, which part can become involved in a lasting relationship with her.

Of course the part that wants her to say "yes" is the physical side of him. It's not very dependable and makes a poor basis for a lasting relationship at any age.

The part that wants her to say "no" is probably all the rest of him.

THE BOYS AND THE GIRLS

"How can I say 'no' and still have friends?"

That depends on the kind of friends you want. No, that's not a very helpful answer, is it? I suppose what I mean is, that kind of "friend" may not be a friend at all. He could be extremely selfish. He wants what *he* wants, even though it may not be a good thing for you at all.

A great deal has been said about what is wrong with physical intimacy among teen-agers. We've talked about the health hazards, the disease problem. We've talked about how difficult it is for the very young to obtain and use contraceptives properly. We've talked about the excellent chance a teen-age girl has of becoming pregnant, and about problems like abortion that go along with that.

There is, however, one thing we haven't mentioned very much, and that is what being promiscuous does to a girl emotionally.

Suppose you are going with a boy and you are madly in love with him. You believe he loves you, too, and that he will be true. You think that whatever the two of you want to do together will be all right, because you really care for each other and someday you will be getting married. So you say "yes" to him.

Time passes, and gradually you find you don't feel quite the same way about each other any more. Your physical intimacy has put a strain on your relationship which you never expected. Maybe you have become jealous of him. You feel that you belong to him now, so that means he belongs to you, and you get terribly upset if he so much as looks at another girl.

This bothers him. He's getting tired of the whole bit.

He's tired of being obligated to spend all his spare time with you, whether he's in the mood or not. He wants out. You have, in effect, lost the friend you were trying so hard to keep. And you have lost even more than that.

Now that the two of you aren't happy together, your reason for being intimate with him doesn't look like such a good reason after all. Your relationship has not been a lasting one. You won't be getting married someday after all. Not only that, but you begin to hear rumors that he is going out with another girl now. Before long you know it's true. Everytime you see them together you wonder if it is that way with them. You're sure it is, and that makes you just one of a series. Now you feel cheap. You feel *used*.

So when another boy comes along, it doesn't take you very long to say yes to him. After all, you have to show the first boy you can get someone else, too, and besides, now you are lonelier than you ever were before boy number one came along. You might as well have the new boy for a friend. If you say yes to him often enough, you'll be able to keep him for awhile.

The one thing you can't seem to keep any more is your self-respect. That's a tragedy, because human beings just can't function properly without a feeling of personal value. You've got to believe in yourself in order to tackle the curriculum you want for the career you are planning. You've got to have some sense of self-worth in order to be pleasant to have around. You've got to have a little self-confidence just to get yourself up in the morning.

You were gradually attaining some self-confidence all the years you were growing up. Now you've lost it all again. You have to start all over again from scratch,

THE BOYS AND THE GIRLS

figuring out who you are and what you are good for. Although they didn't plan it, the boys who were supposed to have been your *friends* have done this to you. And you let them.

"What are you supposed to do if you just can't find a guy who wants a 'nice' girl? So many boys take you out and as soon as they find you won't play their way, they just drop you. The 'good' girls are the ones who sit home every weekend listening to their radios while the C. P.'s have all the dates."

You'll have to fill me in on that "C. P."

"That means a girl who is a common prostitute."

I see. Well, because I am convinced that girls do not understand the physical side of a boy's nature and how strong his urges are, I keep stressing that aspect of boys. But that is by no means all there is to the species, and a girl who appeals solely to that part of a boy usually isn't capable of holding his interest for long. The girl who is a tramp may win the first few battles, but the other kind of girl is really going to win the war.

Boys have minds, too. The most attractive boys usually have very good minds. Once in a while this kind of boy wants a girl he can *talk* to. Not only that, but he wants a girl he can feel proud of in public. Having the other guys envy him because his date makes a good appearance increases his status socially. In addition, he likes a girl who is fun to be with someplace other than in the back seat. He needs someone who can make him laugh and take an interest in his ideas, someone who can help him forget the test he just flunked or the big argument he had with his dad. A girl whose only asset is her willingness to go all the way falls down on all these other counts, don't you see?

In the first place, all the other guys know what she is. Getting a date with her is no triumph at all. You can be pretty sure she can't talk intelligently on any subject. If she could, she wouldn't need to use sex in order to be popular. And even if she did try to make conversation, would he listen to her? You can also be pretty sure the fellow is not eager to invite her home for dinner, and he probably isn't keen about taking her to a big dance or to the rock'n'roll shows with the high-priced tickets. Why spend money on a girl like that? The only exception to all of this is the boy who is interested in absolutely nothing but sex, and that kind of boy has more problems than you'd want to cope with anyway.

But let's get back to the attractive guy with the good mind. What makes him go for a tramp like that? He is experimenting, that's all. And for him the experiment always fails. All it takes is time, usually just long enough for boredom to develop. During that process, the nice girl's greatest asset is the cheap girl herself. Believe it or not, she is working for you.

In her heart she knows what she is and what she has to do to get dates and, unless she is actually retarded, she feels miserable about it inside. Her feelings don't show most of the time. You see her giggling over the notes the boys pass to her in studyhall; you see the fellows waiting for her after school; it looks like a great life. But catch sight of her when she doesn't think anyone is

THE BOYS AND THE GIRLS

looking. Her face, unguarded, will show you it's really a lonely life and a sad one.

The director of a large reform school for girls told me that many of her charges were there, not because they were underprivileged, but because no matter what kind of a home they came from, somewhere along the line they had developed the idea that they were worthless human beings. Maybe a mother habitually treated them like dirt, or maybe a step-father or some other adult abused them physically.

A child may not reason his feelings into words, but the conviction grows in him that if his mother doesn't even *want* him, or his step-father feels free to beat him all the time, he must not be any *good*.

A boy acts out this concept of himself by stealing and committing acts of violence—a girl behaves like a prostitute. Why doesn't the girl react in the same way the boy does? The answer relates to something very deep in the nature of the female. A state welfare department official, who had many years of experience in the handling of juvenile offenders, put it to me this way: When boys in a reform school rebel, they express their feelings through violent destruction of their surroundings; but when girls in a training school rebel, they hurt *themselves*. They bang themselves against the walls, try to jump out of the windows, and slash their wrists. While the boy acts out the deep-rooted conviction that he is a worthless human being by committing crimes, the girl acts out the same conviction by trying to destroy herself. So the tramp or "C.P." in your class may be literally punishing herself for what she thinks she is, and the more she does it, the worse she feels about herself—so the more she does it.

We all have moments of self-doubt, especially during adolescence. Just because you wake up some morning feeling nasty and unloved and wondering what in the world is the matter with you, this doesn't put you in the category with the troubled girls I have been talking about. Those thoughts just mean you are a typical teen-ager. Self-doubt of that sort is all part of the package when you are growing up. But the girl who habitually copes with her feelings of inferiority by going around all four bases on every date has a problem you do not want.

Sure, I know where that leaves *you*. It leaves you home listening to the radio. But suppose you had a chance to be a good friend to one of those very troubled girls. Wouldn't you encourage her to succeed at something else? Wouldn't you encourage her to improve herself in other areas of living? Wouldn't you try to help her gain confidence? Wouldn't you try to inspire her to get better grades or improve her appearance or read a few books some boy might want to talk about sometime?

The same therapy will work for you. While you are waiting for the guys to get around to you, improve yourself. There's always room, isn't there? Think of yourself as a general accumulating war materiel for the time when the last big battles of the war come his way.

Remember this, the boys your age are just as insecure as you are. They try a few go-rounds with the cheap type because they are trying to gain confidence in themselves. No matter how cool they look, they aren't sure of their manhood. They feel a need to prove it, and sex looks like an easy way. They may have no idea you want to go out with them. Your reserve may look like conceit to them.

They need for you to be friendly. Maybe you're not, because you don't want to run after them. Keep on saying "hello" anyway. Don't be a snob either. Just because all but one or two boys in the class look like creeps to you isn't any reason not to be nice. Those creeps are going to turn out to be *men*, believe it or not, and a lot of them are going to turn out to be pretty acceptable men. What they need right now is a friendly smile from a girl who smells sweet, whose hair shines, whose nails are done, and whose blouse is pressed—and who is very clearly not a tramp.

The Marriage Bit

"How can a couple find out if they can be happily married if they don't live together first?"

In other words, what's wrong with trial marriage? Nothing. In those societies where it is an established custom it seems to work pretty well. The two people live together for a period of time and at the end of a year or so they can decide to call the whole thing off, unless the girl is pregnant, in which case they make the arrangement permanent. I wonder, though, what that pregnancy does to them. Suppose they had made up their minds to call it off until the pregnancy came along. Would they resent the baby? At least in a society where trial marriage does not exist, an unhappy marriage does not need to be a baby's fault. The couple go into the marriage knowing that getting out of it again will not be easy.

I suspect that your question really centers on something else, doesn't it? Aren't you saying, how can the couple find out if they are sexually compatible?

"Yes, that's what I meant."

All right, then, let's talk about the feasibility of marriage experiments. Have you ever done experiments in biology or chemistry or physics? If you have, you know that the conditions must be rigidly controlled in order for the experiment to be valid. Our society does not have an approved trial-marriage custom, so it is very difficult to set up the actual conditions for an experimental marriage. Even in a situation where a girl is away from home, attending college, somebody knows where she is. If she has moved in with a fellow in an apartment off-campus, there is always a chance that a relative could drop in, or some acquaintance might gossip, or the dean of women could find out what is going on and call the girl in to talk about it. So this "marriage" lacks something real marriages have—security.

Now security is important. Sexual compatibility often depends upon it. For truly satisfying experiences a woman must feel secure and relaxed and comfortable. At least this is true for most women. So it is possible that in a tense situation a woman would respond to sex in a different way than she would in a secure situation. That means the experiment is not valid. The couple, who might have thought they were completely compatible if they had gone through the actual marriage procedure, could decide they were not meant for each other on the basis of a poor experimental setup.

But let's suppose we could create the proper conditions for a valid test; would that help us to know whether or not a marriage for these two people would work? The answer is, it would not. In the first place, there is a very great deal more to marriage than sexual compatibility. Perhaps we had better pause right here to define that term.

When young people ask a question like yours, it usually means they have a misconception. They have heard a lot of folklore about the relative sizes of the organs involved. The fact is, speaking purely about anatomy and nothing else, physical incompatibility is extremely rare. When it does occur, it can often be treated medically. Historians have told us that Marie Antoinette's husband, Louis XVI, was born with a slight abnormality which made it impossible for him to have normal sex relations. It was operated on and corrected; they had children. So this sort of condition can be treated and, as I said, it is extremely rare.

What we really mean by sexual incompatibility then is not usually physiological but emotional. It is, if you prefer, psychological. And very often it shows up long after the honeymoon is over. It shows up when the couple has gotten deeply in debt, when the husband is working himself to death trying to buy the things the couple wants, when the wife feels overburdened by the care of the home and the children—do you see what I mean? These stresses, these anxieties, affect the couple's sex life. And no relatively carefree trial-marriage period could have provided them with a clear forecast of what was ahead. It might have given warning signs which an experienced marriage counselor could have picked up, but for the couple themselves the warnings might well have been unseen.

You see, the emotional compatibility a couple has is expressed in a satisfying sex life. If they understand one another, if they are kind to one another, if they can help each other over the rough spots, if each of them is genuinely interested in making the other happy, all of this finds expression in their lovemaking. But unfortunately the reverse is not true. Plain physical compatibility will not heal personality conflicts, callousness, ill temper, lack of consideration, and all the other painful aspects of emotional incompatibility. It might be interesting sometime to figure out the comparative time a married couple spends in marketing, looking after the children, caring for the house and yard, eating meals at the table together—and making love.

It's evident then that no trial marriage—not even one that provided the security for a real test of sexual relations—could provide the stresses a married couple lives through over the years in which they are making a home and raising a family.

"Then how can anybody be sure his marriage will work?"

Nobody can. There are some guidelines though. Look sometime at a study of divorce. You will find that certain kinds of marriages have a much higher mortality rate than others. Topping the list are teen-age marriages. An enormous percentage of the marriages of people under the age of nineteen end in divorce. Another hazard is the marriage of couples who come from vastly different cultural backgrounds, particularly mixed-religion marriages. This does not mean that teen-age marriages never work or that marriage between individuals of different faiths never works. It just means those couples have a tougher time. More is required of them—more maturity, more patience, more understanding, more love. And that brings us to another big factor in marriage that an experimental marriage such as our hypothetical case of the girl away at college and living secretly with a boy off-campus would never be able to include: in-laws. You rarely marry an individual. You marry his or her *family*, too.

"Well, suppose a young couple has thought about all these things and has decided to get married with a lot of careful planning. Say they have decided he will finish school first so he can get a good job. They are going to save money so that when they do get married, they can buy what they need. They are going to keep all the in-laws happy and wait and have a big wedding. Now isn't a long engagement a problem, too?"

You mean, sexually?

"Yes. You know, the strain of holding themselves back when they know they love each other—it could make them fight with each other, couldn't it? It could even make the fellow want to go out with somebody else once in a while. Wouldn't it be better if they went ahead and had sex before marriage?"

It might. I won't argue with you about that. The sort of couple you are describing seems pretty mature. College age, I assume. So I would go along with you on that and say that by the time young people are out of their teens they ought to be able to make a decision like that. And some studies that have been made seem to point to a trend in that direction—premarital sex during the engagement period. Some authorities see this as a harmful course,

THE MARRIAGE BIT

while others claim that the marriage which follows that sort of an engagement is in no way handicapped by the premarital sex. But engagements are broken more easily than marriages are. There is always the question, what if something goes wrong? If the marriage does not take place, what then? Will the girl feel worse about the ending of that kind of an engagement than she would about the ending of the old-fashioned kind? And what about the fellow? Would he feel more obligated, more guilty about any misgivings he develops?

"I don't see why the age of the people matters. If people in their twenties can do something, why can't people in their teens? I know sixteen-and seventeen-year-olds who have more common sense than some others who are a few years older."

Well, there must be some reason why more teen-age marriages fail. There must be something different about a large number of sixteen-and seventeen-year-olds. What do you people think it might be?

"Kids aren't sure what they want. You like one fellow, or one kind of girl, and then you like another. You are still finding out what you really want."

That's a good point. What are some other differences?

"I think teen-agers want to have a good time. They haven't had a chance to do everything they want to do yet, but when you are in college or out working on a job and have your own money to spend, you can do everything you want."

So you are saying that a person who is a little older is more ready to settle down. Yes, that's right. Often when very young people get married, they begin to feel they have missed a lot, and they want to go out with other people after awhile. Let's think about the *reasons* for getting married. What motivates a couple in their twenties to marry, and what motivates a couple in their teens to marry? Is it the same?

"To get away from home. I think a lot of kids, especially girls who have a rough time at home, want to get away. But if a girl is working, if she's older, she could have a place of her own. So if she gets married, it must be because she really wants to."

"Don't a lot of couples get married because they are going to have a baby?"

Yes, that's true. And certainly the couple who is older has a better chance of dealing with the challenge of establishing a home for themselves and their child than the very young couple. We all know the effect the amount of education you have has on the kind of job you will find. So we can see already those stresses and strains we spoke about—the ones that provide the real test of a marriage.

"And the in-law problem would be worse, too. If the teen-age girl's parents hate the boy for getting her pregnant, they could make her give up the baby instead of getting married, couldn't they? And they could still tell her what to do all the time because she is a minor?"

Now you are getting into questions a lawyer should answer. The laws are different in different states, and you would have to look them up. Generally, though, I think a married teen-ager is considered an adult. The term used in court is "emancipated." No matter what the girl's age

THE MARRIAGE BIT

is, nobody can make her give up her baby. She must sign the papers herself, even if she is very young, even if she isn't married.

"But you can't get married without your parents' consent, can you?"

In the states I know about, you can if a baby is expected. You must get proof from the doctor that the girl is pregnant, and then you can get a marriage license. The question for us to consider is, is it a good idea to get married at an early age?

"Well, if you are going to have a baby, you **have** *to."*

No, you don't. That's the point. A minister I know does a lot of work with young people, and he has told me that he always insists that young people who are thinking about getting married because a baby is expected clearly understand this. He tells them, "Nobody *has* to get married. There are alternatives. So if you do get married, don't ever throw this pregnancy up to the other party later. Nobody can make you get married. There is no law that can make you get married. Don't ever tell anybody you *had* to get married. If you don't intend to do right by the other person, getting married now will only make matters worse." So the decision as to whether or not it is a good idea to get married for a particular couple at a particular time must rest on something other than pregnancy or a desire to get away from home. What should the decision rest on?

Love, shouldn't it?

And how would you define love?

BETTER THAN THE BIRDS—SMARTER THAN THE BEES

"Love is when you care more about the other person than you do about yourself."

Good. So the person who says to you, "If you love me, you'll do what *I* want," doesn't love you. That is selfishness. In view of the problems which every marriage must face wouldn't you agree that even in marriages which begin under the best possible circumstances genuine, unselfish affection is a must? If you have that, then you can tackle the other problems.

"Well, if marriage is so difficult, isn't it wrong for the magazines and the movies to make it all seem so—I don't know."

Romantic? They make marriage look like a happy ending, don't they, instead of just the beginning. Yes, it is wrong. It gives young people all sorts of wrong ideas. Then when the first real trouble comes along in a marriage, they are ready to give up. They expect a fairy-tale existence, based on the magazine and TV ads of the happy family in their beautiful home, brushing their teeth together and laughing. The fact is, marriage takes work just as anything worthwhile takes work. If you want to learn to play the guitar or to swim a mile or to get into college or to lose fifteen pounds, you fully expect to work at it. But after the wedding bells ring, you are shocked to find that you are not automatically living happily ever after. Maybe your generation can do better. Maybe you have seen so much on television and in real life that you are not as likely to swallow the Hollywood mythology. I hope so.

Briarpatch Children

"Everybody says that girls shouldn't mess around because they might get pregnant, but that argument always strikes me as sort of silly, because I really can't imagine me getting pregnant."

That's what the girls in homes for unwed mothers always say. They will tell you they just never dreamed it could happen to them. Hearing them, I am reminded of the lemmings. Have you ever heard about the lemmings? The poet John Masefield wrote a sonnet about them; maybe you have read it in English class. They are little mouselike animals who live in the northern hemisphere, especially in the mountains of Scandinavia. Every five, or ten, or sometimes twenty years, they come rushing out of their homes and make a mad dash toward the sea. When they get there, they plunge in and drown themselves. Nobody knows why. It is just some instinct that drives them to do it.

We don't know exactly how many girls get pregnant out of wedlock every year in this country. A large number of them get married before the birth takes place. Others give a married name on the birth certificate to conceal the illegitimacy. And of course we have no idea how many illegal abortions are performed. We are pretty sure that unmarried girls get pregnant at least 500,000 times a year, and maybe it's more like a million times a year. One study estimated that an illegitimate baby is born to a young girl every two-and-one-half minutes.

So you see why I think of the lemmings when I hear a girl say, "It just couldn't happen to me." A girl like that is simply closing her eyes to the facts, to the danger, and plunging blindly on toward a sort of self-destruction, almost as though she is being driven by some mysterious impulse.

My mother says only poor people who live in bad neighborhoods have illegitimate babies. She says they do it mostly to get more money from the welfare agencies. But in my class at school—not my homeroom, you know, but my grade—three girls have gone away, and the kids are saying the girls are pregnant. I don't know whether to believe it or not."

I don't either, but I can tell you definitely that poor people in what you call bad neighborhoods are not the only ones having illegitimate babies. While we are at it, let me correct that idea about welfare. The additional money for another baby in our state will barely buy the baby's milk. It will not pay for a crib or baby clothes or diapers or anything else. And there's a law setting the maximum amount that any one family can get. That means that the welfare check does not increase beyond a certain point, no matter how many children you have. So a family with six or eight or ten or twelve children must live on a check the same size as a family with four children would get. Take my word for it, nobody has babies for the welfare money.

To answer the rest of your questions we must depend on bits and pieces of information. Women's colleges, for example, give evidence that there are a large number of abortions taking place—not on the campus, of course, but during vacations from school the girls who can afford it go away somewhere for the operation. I have to use vague terms like "a large number" because this information comes from off-the-record talks with faculty members who are close to some of the students. Ministers who work at churches in upper-income neighborhoods report that more and more families are coming to them for advice because they have a teen-ager in this kind of trouble. The homes for unwed mothers are full, and most of them are working on plans to expand their facilities. Of course, poor people do not send their daughters there. The girls in homes for pregnant girls are from middle- and upper-income families. So even though we have very few clear statistics on this problem, we can say pretty definitely that it is a problem which affects every neighborhood and every school and not just the homes of the poorly educated and the unemployed.

"Why can't girls from poor families go to homes for unwed mothers?"

They can. It costs money, of course, but there are social agencies that will help a girl whether she has any money or not. The main reason that girls from poorer families do not go into homes for unwed mothers is that they do not have the same need to. In a better-income neighborhood, having a baby when you are not married is a great disgrace. It must be concealed. The baby must be born in secret and given up for adoption so that the girl can come back home as though it never happened; she will say she spent the time at her grandmother's, or something. But in a neighborhood where family troubles are common, where the man on this corner drinks, and the man across the street has been out of work for months, and the woman across the alley was deserted by her husband, and your friend's older sister cannot afford a divorce so she is living with another man anyway—in this kind of neighborhood, having a baby out of wedlock is not such a shocking thing. The girl can stay home until time for the baby to be born, and after the baby is born, she can bring it home from the hospital, and the neighbors will come in and admire it.

"It happened to someone I know, and I felt so sorry for her. She came from a nice family and, like you said, she had to hide her condition. She went to a Home in another city, and then she signed papers to give the baby away. I was the only one who knew about it except her family. She wrote me when she was in the hospital, and she said her baby was so beautiful. After she came home she cried and cried because she missed the baby. I don't think she'll ever get over it. I don't think it's fair. If she had been poor, she wouldn't have had to give her baby up. She could have kept it and not needed to go through all that sadness."

BRIARPATCH CHILDREN

I understand what you are saying about your friend, and it is a very sad thing. I can't go along with you when you say she will never "get over it," because she will. The grief will subside in time. And she is surely a much wiser and more mature person now, isn't she? So the experience has changed her; it has not left her where it found her. Certainly, she will never forget her baby, not even when she marries and has other children. A young woman I knew, who went through that experience and later married a fine young man and had other children, told me her first baby had a little birthmark on his ankle and that she found herself looking for that mark whenever she saw a group of children. Two years after it had happened, she was watching the toddlers in the sandbox in the park. Six years afterward, she was watching the first graders lining up to get on the school bus. She felt though that she had done the right thing. She said she had decided it would have been selfish for her to keep the baby. She couldn't give him a good home—not then, anyway—except by giving him up. That was her way of giving him a good home.

Because, you see, that girl from a poor neighborhood, even though she is spared the anguish of parting from her child in his infancy, does not have an easy time of it later on. Neither does the child. He is still, regardless of the neighborhood he grows up in, a "briarpatch child." That's what they used to be called in olden times, and they are still called by that name in the southern mountain country. The name says a great deal. It indicates a child born secretly, in the wilds. It means a child who is different from other children, and who is handicapped by the ill-luck of his birth. Times have changed a great deal but not enough for the briarpatch child to have the same chance for a happy life that the child born of married parents will have.

"You just said something different from what you said awhile ago. First you said it isn't as much of a disgrace in a neighborhood where there are a lot of problems, and then you said an unwed mother from that kind of a neighborhood still has a hard time and so does her child."

All right, let's straighten that out.

The sort of thing we call a "social stigma"—a bad mark against you, something people can gossip about—is not so severe in a neighborhood where out-of-wedlock pregnancies are more common. The other adverse factors surrounding the child and his family will, however, still be severe and, in some instances, worse.

First, let's talk about families. In other cultures families are very different from the family as we know it in this country today. Take, for example, the typical old Chinese family you read about in the writings of novelist Pearl Buck. The young man marries and brings his wife home to live with his mother and father. There are also in the household the young man's older brothers and their wives. His sisters who have married have gone to live as members of their husbands' families. But there are younger, unmarried sisters still at home, and aged grandparents, and maybe an unmarried aunt. And there are the children of the older brothers. Everybody lives and works together. The men and the younger women work the farm, while the older women keep house, prepare the meals, and look after the little children. The old people make the decisions. The younger ones do as they are told. There is no rigid distinction made between my children and your children, my mother and your mother. So if one of the young mothers should fall ill and die, or if one of the young fathers should have to go away to war, there is still the family. There is still security for a child; there are still plenty of people to look after him.

Now I don't need to tell you how different our family life is. The first thing a young married couple wants to do is get a little place of their own. The newspaper advice columns are filled with letters from daughters who complain that their mothers or mothers-in-law keep trying to tell them how to raise their children, and from mothers and mothers-in-law who disapprove of the way their grandchildren are being raised. When an older relative needs care, we find it necessary to send him or her to a nursing home. Our houses are too small to hold several generations. We pride ourselves on our independence and our right to do as we please.

What happens though when a young girl brings home to her mother a "briarpatch child"? The question at once arises, "Who is going to be mother to this baby?" Particularly in a home where there is very little money, this question must come up. Will daughter go back to school and try to complete her education while grandmother keeps the baby? Or will the baby's grandmother continue working at the job she has held for a long time so that her daughter must drop out of school to raise the baby? In that case, will the daughter try to continue her education at night? If she does, what will her mother say? Will she say, "I have worked hard all day, and I'm not going to baby-sit at night?" Or will she say, "All right, I will keep the baby the nights you go to school, but don't think you are going out on weekends, because you are not." This means that the teen-age girl, who has barely begun to have the good times most of you can look forward to, is going to be forced to sit home with her baby night after night while other people her own age are going to parties. Or it means that life in the home will consist of constant fights about whether or not the girl should go out or stay home.

Then there is the financial question. Can the young mother support her baby? Even if the child's natural father can give five dollars a week, or maybe ten, will this be enough? Or will her parents be feeding and clothing the child? If they do, will they not feel they have a right to decide how the child will be raised? The fact that the young mother made a mess of her life leads us to suspect she was not happy with her own upbringing and family life. Will she want her mother to make the same mistakes with another child? If she does not, what can she do about it? She hasn't the money to move away. Her social life is severely limited by her responsibilities. Boys that she does get to see know all about her; they are probably going to want the same thing the father of her baby got. Her chances of meeting the kind of a young man who will marry her and make a home for her baby are almost nil.

What sort of a young man would it take, and what would be required of him? It would take a young man who loved her so much that her past didn't matter to him. We must assume the baby's father has removed himself from the picture. If he had cared for her deeply, she probably would not be in the spot she is in. So the Mr. Right she is hoping for will have to face the prospect of raising another man's child as his own. He must face the possibility that the child will look like the other man and that the child may remind the wife of her first love. She probably hates him now, but the young man who marries her cannot be sure of this. He must ask himself, "Can I love this child?" There are very few young men who feel they can take on this kind of a job.

What of the child? His young life begins with a large share of built-in and almost unavoidable confusion in regard to his identity and his status in society. Take this young woman who holds him, who is she? She loves him, but she is not the one who buys him things; the older woman does that. The young woman calls the older woman "Mom." Shall he call the older woman "Mom," too? And does that mean the younger woman is his sister? When he falls and hurts himself, he may run to the older woman, because she seems to know more. When he does, however, the younger one is hurt. Why is this? And what about his father? The other children have someone to call "Daddy." When he asks questions, he is told his daddy went away; or maybe he is told his daddy lives several blocks away and may be seen going past the house in a car once in a while.

We do not know what this does to a child. There are some facts which lead us to believe it has a very bad effect. One of these facts relates to teen-age crime. The greatest proportion of juvenile delinquency comes from homes where there is no father.

Again we do not know what this situation does to the young mother. We have some statistics which lead us to believe it has a very bad effect. Studies have shown that the young girl who goes into a home for unwed mothers and gives her baby up for adoption almost never gets into that situation again. On the other hand, the girl who stays at home and keeps her baby has a strong chance of having another illegitimate child within two years of the first one.

It seems incredible that any girl above the lowest level on the intelligence scale would let herself get into all that heartache again, but when you stop to think about it, the reasons are not hard to find. She has all the same problems she had before—the problems that made it possible for her to get into trouble the first time—only now, she has additional problems as well. Her relationship with her family is under greater strain. She has money troubles. Her social life is hampered by the baby. She is probably lonelier than ever. And she may be desperately looking for a way out, a man to marry her. Her education may have come to a complete stop. She may face a life almost devoid of hope.

The girl who has gone into a home for unwed mothers comes out of her experience with a lot of plus factors. Chances are she has had skilled psychological help during the period she awaited the birth and during the critical period between the birth and the signing of the adoption papers. Nothing will allay the anguish of giving up her child, and I do not mean to minimize that aspect of the situation. Unless you have held your own newborn baby in your arms, you will not be able to imagine what it means to relinquish a child. Nevertheless, the girl who has gone through this experience with the help of experienced counselors should have learned a great deal about herself. She should have learned why this happened to her. She should have grown enough so that it cannot happen again. She goes back to her life pretty much where she left it, with school and social life ahead of her again. Inside, of course, she is different; but if her arrangements have remained secret, no one will know why.

"Then you are saying that when this happens to a girl, going away and giving her baby up is the right answer?"

No. The only right answer is not to get pregnant out of wedlock. Once a girl is pregnant out of wedlock, her answers boil down to a choice between lesser evils. It is better to marry the teen-age father of your baby than to have a criminal abortion. It may be better to stay home than to marry a boy who doesn't love you very much and cannot make a home for you. It is better to go away to a home for pregnant girls than to stay home and let your problems multiply. And in between these choices, others are beginning to open up. There are some public schools where the pregnant girl can continue her education and get experienced help, even though she remains at home.

None of the possible ways of handling the problem is perfect. Even if you had the money to travel three thousand miles away to the most beautifully equipped Home in the country, there is always a chance that your situation will be found out. Some friend may talk. The boy may talk. Someone may see you on your way to the doctor. There is no perfect solution except prevention of the problem.

Another factor enters in. There was a time when the demand for babies for adoption was very great. Now many couples who formerly could not have children are being treated with new methods. There are even fertility clinics to help them. So there are fewer couples now who can have families in no other way but through adoption. And the supply of available babies is obviously increasing all the time. There are a great many babies born with no hope of adoption. For example, the supply of Negro babies far exceeds the demand for them. Children of mixed racial heritage, such as the offspring of American soldiers and Korean or Japanese or Vietnamese women, have almost no hope of finding homes. Every adoptive infant is supposed to be perfect, too. That means if an unmarried girl gives birth to a child with a defect, a heart murmur or some malformation which cannot be completely corrected, her baby may never be adopted.

"What happens to a child like that?"

Sometimes the girl's family decides to keep the baby, or place it in an institution themselves. Sometimes the child remains in foster care all his growing-up years. There are very few orphanages, as we used to know them. Attempts are made to place children in individual homes wherever possible. There are not nearly enough good ones. Social agencies and welfare departments always need many more foster parents than they have, and children who grow up in foster care are, unfortunately, moved from place to place a great deal. Now can you see why social workers like me are not simply being negative and restrictive when we insist that children who cannot be cared for must not be brought into the world? We see what happens to these children. Our hearts are broken by the sight, over and over again.

"I know what you say is true about the parents in the suburbs, but I think kids themselves are changing. A girl I know had to go away, and nearly all the kids were on her side. One boy made a remark about her, and the other boys roughed him up. A couple of the kids went to see her teachers to get them to send her schoolwork home; and when our English teacher asked why they were doing this, they said because it could have happened to them."

I am glad to hear that. Surely, the girl in trouble needs all the help and support and understanding she can get. And it is certainly true that it could have happened to dozens of others. Shunning the girl in trouble is narrow-minded and prejudiced and belongs back in the Puritan days when witches were hanged and people were put in the stocks for swearing "Upon my word!" Maybe you can help the parents see that.

"I know a girl who was gone the whole last half of the year, and I think she went away to have a baby. At least there were a lot of rumors. She seems awfully lonely this year, and I'd like to be friends with her, but I don't know what to say."

Surely you would say nothing about the rumors. You would approach her with an obvious desire to be friends with her for herself. You see, the girl who has to go away to have a baby has months in which to wonder about herself, about what kind of a girl she is and why this happened to her. The fact is, she is not different from other girls. In homes for unwed mothers and in schools for pregnant students you will find pretty girls and plain girls and bright girls and slow girls and sweet girls and catty girls—they are all just girls. Often they are not the most promiscuous girls in their crowd, by any means. The really promiscuous girl generally does not become pregnant. There are many instances where the girl who has gotten pregnant went with only one boy and thought she loved him very much. There are even cases where a girl made the mistake of accepting a ride home with a crowd of boys she didn't know very well, was attacked, and became pregnant from that single experience. So the girl who has had a baby out of wedlock is just like the girls who have not except, perhaps, that her luck was bad.

Her feelings of embarrassment and inferiority may be much greater than those of other girls. She needs your friendship—and your tact—very much.

"Does anybody know why girls get pregnant? We know about the biology, but—because we are getting the facts about the biology, girls ought to know better, don't you think?"

Well, there is a lot of the lemming impulse we talked about earlier, the devil-may-care attitude that it couldn't possibly happen to me. I suspect that there is a very great deal of concern under the surface of that seeming heedlessness.

BRIARPATCH CHILDREN

Most unmarried mothers have had very poor communication with their parents. They have been unable to talk to their mothers and fathers. They feel the parents will not listen to them, or will misunderstand them, or will give them a very hard time about what they are trying to say.

Often the unmarried mother has not been successful socially. She is rarely one of the most popular girls in her class. This may be why she felt she needed to give a boy everything he wanted in order to keep his attention.

Maybe her loneliness stems from other causes. Sometimes she is the less attractive or less bright sister in the family. Sometimes she is an only child who may have yearned, down deep, for something of her own to love. Quite a few unwed mothers have, for one reason or another, no father. This could lead them to search for love from the opposite sex.

Occasionally, we come across a girl whose mother is very successful, socially or in business. The girl may feel it is hopeless to compete with her mother except in one way: she, too, has the necessary equipment for reproduction. Perhaps the girl has been very much dominated and has had no experience making her own decisions or assuming responsibility on her own. Therefore, when she gets involved with a boy, she, from habit, lets him take over. Unless he plans realistically about the possibility of pregnancy, no preventive steps are taken. When the pregnancy comes along, she is helpless.

Another type of girl is bitterly rebellious about the domination she feels she has experienced at home. Her pregnancy is an unconscious act of defiance. She is going to show her family. She is going to give them something to talk about. She is really going to put them in a spot. Of course the sad part is that whatever suffering she causes her parents is no match for the suffering she causes herself.

So the answer to your question is, there are many reasons why girls get pregnant out of wedlock. Because of the differences in individual girls, the reason for each girl is unique. The job done by the skilled counselor for the unwed mother is designed to help each girl find *her* reason, so that it does not happen again.

"Can't a boy who gets a girl pregnant be taken to court?"

Yes, in a couple of ways. In the case of a very young girl it is possible that a boy can be charged with a crime simply for having had sexual relations with her, whether she has become pregnant or not. This is called "statutory rape." It means that a very young girl—in our state it is a girl under sixteen—is not old enough to know what she is doing. She has not reached what the courts call "the age of consent." So even if she agreed with what the boy was doing, he can be charged, at least technically, with having raped her.

The other way he can be taken to court is on a support proceeding. For this the girl must wait until after the baby has been born. This means she—or her parents—must make the arrangements for her prenatal care and for paying the hospital bill. Then after the baby has been born, the girl must fill out the necessary legal papers, naming the father of the baby. He receives a summons to appear in court where the amount which he must pay can be set up. He can be made to contribute to the child's support until the child becomes of age. If the child should be handicapped in some way, the father could be made to support him as long as he lives. In addition to regular support payments, designed to cover the cost of the child's food, clothing, and shelter, he may have to pay for hospital costs for the child's illnesses. If the child should die, the father may have to pay for the funeral. These support payments can remain in effect even if the girl marries someone else later on.

"What if the boy claims he is not the father?"

Then the girl has a problem. If the boy brings witnesses who swear that they were with her, too, the judge, or whichever officer of the court is handling the hearing, has to try to decide. When there is strong doubt, it would be unfair to saddle the young man with what may very well turn out to be thousands of dollars worth of payments. It is a very serious thing for the young man. If he fails to make payments for which he is obligated by a court order, he can be sent to prison.

"What if he is going to school and doesn't have a job?"

Often the court will continue the case until the young man is in a position to make payments. It would not be logical to make him stop school—he might never get a job. They try to work something out. No matter what arrangements are made, the father of the baby has a heavy burden of responsibility.

"Does it have to go to court? Can't the people make some agreement themselves?"

Yes, they can, except where a social agency or an institution must involve themselves. If a child must be placed in foster care with the department of welfare, a court order is required to ensure that the child will have some support from the parent. An informal arrangement is not good enough in that case.

"If a baby is adopted, do the parents still support it?"

No, once the original expenses are out of the way—the hospital bill, the girl's care in a Home, the baby's care during the period before the mother signs him away— neither the mother nor the natural father has any more responsibility for the child.

"Doesn't the baby's father have to sign the papers, too?"

No. If he has not married the mother, he has no legal say whatever about what will become of the child. He cannot have a say in whether it is adopted or kept, or what its religion will be, or where it will live.

"What if the baby's mother doesn't want the child, but the father does? Suppose his mother, the baby's grandmother, wanted to keep it?"

That would be very difficult, legally. It would almost have to be a complete adoption procedure, just as though a family of total strangers wanted the baby. The baby's natural father has no legal rights to the child at all; all he has is a legal obligation to support the child until he becomes an adult or until he is adopted by someone else.

"Going back to the support hearing—I thought they could prove who the father was with a blood test."

No. They can prove who it wasn't. You see, there are different types of blood. I can't give you the details; it is all highly technical. In brief, if a baby has a certain type of blood and the mother has a certain type of blood, they know what type of blood the father's could be. That means if the young man the girl names as the father has that type of blood, he could be the father. So could all the other men in the world with that blood type. If the young man is trying to get out of supporting the baby, he may bring into the hearing a friend to claim he had been with the girl too. But if the friend has the wrong blood type, the officer of the court may decide that the accused young man must pay the support.

On the other hand, if the accused—or perhaps we should call him by the correct legal name, "the putative father"—if the putative father turns out to have a blood type which could not possibly have gone into making the child's blood, then the test will clear him completely. You can see that it is a very unclear business. There is no absolutely accurate test of fatherhood. Maybe sometime medical science will find one. It certainly would help.

"Where are the homes for unwed mothers?"

You can find out about them by asking anyone whose job it is to help people in trouble. That means your doctor, your clergyman, the school guidance counselor, or any social worker. There are many of these homes. A lot of them fall into three general categories, and you can find them in the telephone book under these names. The

Florence Crittenton Homes are in many cities; they take girls of all kinds. The Catholic Church has many homes of this type, too, and you could learn about them by calling Catholic Charities or whatever the central social agency for the Catholic Church in your area happens to be. The Salvation Army also maintains homes for pregnant girls, you could call your nearest Salvation Army Office to find where their homes are. If you get completely lost, there is a department of welfare in every state, every county, and every city of any size. It may take a few phone calls, but someone is sure to have the information you need. Finally, there is your public library. Don't be bashful about asking the librarian for help. She doesn't need to know you are not doing a term paper on unwed mothers.

"If a girl doesn't want the family doctor or her mother to know, where can she go to find out if she is pregnant?"

Almost nowhere. This whole area of medical care for minors is under exhaustive examination now. It is a big question. The law generally is very specific; no minor can be treated without the consent of a parent or legal guardian.* This means that if a child gets a broken arm on the school playground and is taken to a hospital by the school nurse, the hospital cannot set the bone until the boy's mother is found. Now in a case like that waiting is not serious. It protects the patient and his family; it ensures their right to have the medical work done by a doctor of their own choosing. Also, it is a safeguard for

* The laws dealing with treatment of minors are undergoing revision in some states.

religious freedom, since there are some religions which oppose medical attention or which have restrictions on the kind of medical attention they will accept.

There are other cases, however, which cause doctors grave concern. These are the cases when an emergency operation is needed, and the patient and the surgical team wait while the police go around in squad cars looking for the child's parents to get them to sign a paper. Often where there has been an accident involving young people, the emergency treatment is given anyway. But hospitals are understandably concerned about this—they could be sued.

You can see why they are not going to break the rules for a girl who is pregnant. She has time. They probably will not turn her down cold. Someone will talk with her and point out to her the need to bring her mother in. Her mother is going to find out anyway, if she really is pregnant. The same thing is true for the teen-ager who wants medical treatment because of a suspected case of venereal disease. The medical people do not want to turn you away. They want to help you. You may happen to find one who will risk breaking the law because he wants so much to help. But it is much kinder and wiser, on your part, to go about it the right way. Tell your parents, and have one of them take you for the checkup.

We have one more question. It says: *"How can I tell my mother I am going to have a baby?"*

My dear, I wish I knew. If you go to your clergyman or your guidance counselor or another relative, your mother will surely say, "Why didn't you tell me first?" She is going to be hurt and upset, no matter how you go about it. So are you. I believe your own greatest suffering will stem from delay, because you are not only thinking of yourself and what you must go through, but you are thinking of her and how she will feel, aren't you? Why not begin with this? Tell her that the last thing you want to do is hurt her, because you love her very much. Say that you are going to have to hurt her now, because you need her now more than you have ever needed her in your whole life. Then put your arms around her, and tell her.

Don't wait. Do it right away. And remember, there are lots of us waiting to help.

You and the No-No's

"When I try to talk to my mother about sex, she says there is only one thing I need to know—the commandment which says 'Thou shalt not commit adultery.' She says it's God's law, and if I break it, he will punish me. Then I pick up a magazine and read that some theologians say that God is dead. How am I supposed to know what to think?"

When you say that, you make me think about the television comedy skit about Adam and Eve. Every time they went near the tree of knowledge, this terrible deep voice from offstage boomed out, "THAT'S A NO-NO!" Perhaps an audience of very simple, very primitive people would have been terrified; but the audience in the television studio thought it was very funny, and so did the people in my living room. Perhaps we thought it was funny because we know we are not children any more. We know that our thirst for knowledge will not be quenched by our being told to stop seeking it. What this shows about us is what a long way we have come, and the attitude of your mother and others of her generation shows how fast we have made the trip.

It wasn't very long ago that people believed it was wicked to talk about sex. When Sigmund Freud began talking about sex two or three generations ago, everyone was simply scandalized. The Victorians believed that the sole purpose of sex was to make babies. The thought that it might be a way of expressing love—or worse, that it might actually be fun—would have horrified them.

That is why until very recently your mother's answer was perfectly acceptable. Fear of God was the deterrent that kept people from stealing and committing adultery and killing one another. At least it kept a lot of people from doing those things. They were not good, mind you, out of love for their fellow men. They were good because they did not want to go to hell. Life for them was a path picked carefully between all the great, booming No-No's, with eternal damnation lurking all around the borders of the path. Now we have come of age. We are not afraid of the tree of knowledge. Good or bad, we yearn to taste of it. If the "death-of-God" theologians have helped us reach this point, we should be grateful to them.

However, they have left us about where we were. Those of us who did not believe before are continuing not to believe, and those of us who always have believed are going on believing.

There is one difference. Those of us who do believe have had to stop giving pat answers and stock phrases for everything. We have had to find the real rock-bottom wisdom behind our beliefs and spell it out. We have had

YOU AND THE NO-NO'S

to grope our way toward a code of ethics that is honest and realistic and which is based upon a clear recognition of our own needs as human beings and the needs of our fellow human beings. In short, we have had to stop saying "The reason you must not do that is because it's a No-No." Personally, I think that was what God intended for us to do all along.

"My mother won't even go so far as to talk about that commandment. The first time I asked her what adultery was, she said you weren't supposed to sell milk with a lot of water in it. Why are adults so embarrassed when they have to talk about sex?"

Because they just aren't used to it. Most of the people in the generation ahead of you never got any sex education at all, except the kind you pick up in jokes. If they know the names for things, they have probably never said them aloud. Even if a parent goes to the library and gets a book on the subject, it is difficult to talk about it, particularly to his or her own child. One mother told me, "I can't talk about it because I'm afraid my daughter will start to wonder about her father and *me.*" I know this seems unbelievable to you, but it's true, and you're going to have to be patient with your parents.

"A girl I know got married because she had to, and the school agreed to let her finish high school; but the parents of the other kids had a meeting and signed a petition to make her quit because they didn't want their children to see a pregnant girl in school."

BETTER THAN THE BIRDS—SMARTER THAN THE BEES

If that's the way the parents feel, they had better not let their children out of the house.

Aren't you glad times are changing? I am. You people are going to do so much better.

"I think a lot of middle-aged people who are so holier-than-thou are really mad because they aren't having as much fun as teen-agers are today."

A writer took care of people like that a long time ago. His name was H. G. Wells, and he defined moral indignation as "Jealousy—with a halo."

Seriously, you must not misinterpret the adult concern. Much of it is fear for your safety and well-being. Maybe you don't read the papers, but the older generation does. Every case of death from a criminal abortion, or the rape of a girl who was parked with her date on a lonely road, makes your parents worry about *you*. And it isn't foolish. It is very well-founded concern.

"But parents have such artificial ways of judging. I could bring a full-fledged sex maniac into the house, and if he had a haircut, they would think he was a charming boy. But as soon as they see a guy with hair over his collar, they are absolutely convinced he is addicted to heroin and runs a teen-age white-slavery ring."

Don't you do the same thing? When a substitute walks in the schoolroom with her skirt halfway to her ankles, don't you make up your mind she is a complete freak?

"In one of my classes the teacher was talking about a book he had read that said there are some times when it may be more right to break a commandment than to

keep it. He told about cases where you had to spy for your country and get information. It was called—I forget the name."

That is usually called "situation ethics." It simply means that each situation has its own unique moral implications, and you cannot make a rule ahead of time that will be infallibly right for every situation. As you say, a spy in the service of his country might need to break a lot of commandments to get information. A soldier is ordered to break the rule, "Thou shalt not kill." Was your question, "Is situation ethics right or wrong?"

"Not exactly. I wasn't thinking about war, anyway. I'm pretty sure if you are serving your country you need to do what you are told. I was thinking about sex and kids my age. It seems to me the situation is different today, and what may have been wrong in the past might be right now. I mean, if you aren't being selfish, if you just want to make someone happy, couldn't you call it 'loving your neighbor'?"

Sometimes it helps to think of immoral behavior as a *mistake*. In fact, one definition of sin is "missing the mark." Moral behavior, on the other hand, is that behavior which experience has proved will work best in the long run. For example, $2 + 2 = 5$ is a mistake. It is "wrong." It is also very inconvenient. It makes a mess of the checkbook stubs. You have to go back and do everything over, because $2 + 2 = 5$ simply doesn't work out right.

The behavior that society generally condemns has a similar effect. If you talk about dope, you are speaking of a mistake that leads to addiction, to bondage. Excessive and improper use of alcohol leads to accidents, loss of employment, and, ultimately, to body and brain damage. When we come to your question, we must say that the bulk of our experience points to the fact that premarital sex generally has some bad or at least some inconvenient results. Even if we can find a way around the health hazards and the risk of out-of-wedlock pregnancy, there are the subtle psychological factors. What does it do to your concept of yourself? The writer Ernest Hemingway, who certainly was no square, said, "What is moral is what you feel good after and what is immoral is what you feel bad after." Expand that word "after" to include, not just a minute after, but a month or six months after, and you have a very good definition. How are you going to feel a year from now if that girl, who may have had no experience until she became so fond of you, has become a complete pig? It may not happen that way, but you will never know, really, what effect you have had on her and on her life.

You see, the real moral disease of our times is not sexual promiscuity or graft in government or crookedness in business or organized crime. It is "What's in it for me"? That is what lies behind all the evils you can mention. To be frank, in my judgment that is what lies behind your question.

You say you are not being selfish—you just want to make somebody happy—and you ask if that kind of premarital sex isn't "loving your neighbor." It seems to me that if your real, genuine motive is to make that girl happy, you would be giving some thought to marrying her. The fact is, girls in your age-group are not primarily interested in their sex drives. They are interested in love. The test of love is never sex; it is serious, long-range intentions.

All right, I know your answer to that. You are too young to think about getting married. That is probably true. If it is, I suggest you give consideration to the thought that maybe you are also too young for sexual relations. I say that because I believe if you are honest, you will admit that the kind of sex you have in mind is selfish sex, and selfish sex—at any age—is immoral. Unselfish sex involves a willingness to make a deep personal commitment. It involves a willingness to give something of yourself other than the glands and the hormones. It involves a willingness to engage in a complete relationship, a relationship which includes the total person of each of the partners. The way this sort of relationship, this sort of commitment, is usually expressed is through marriage.

"*Usually,*" I say. Note that I am not making the blanket statement that all sex outside of marriage is wrong and all sex inside of marriage is right. There are some terribly selfish married people, and this is immoral. On the other hand, it may be possible for two mature individuals to have a very complete, very unselfish relationship without marriage. They would need, however, to be very mature indeed, because an arrangement like that includes a great deal of built-in doubt and insecurity. They would have to be old enough and wise enough to make no demands upon one another and trust each other completely.

Very young people just aren't emotionally equipped for this kind of relationship. They are too unsure of themselves and each other. The girl, particularly, needs the security of marriage or engagement or at least being engaged to become engaged; and even those last two leave a lot to be desired. This is why I say that if you are genuinely unselfish in your regard for the girl, you will express this by a willingness to consider a more complete commitment or, failing that, to postpone the sexual relationship until later.

Why should this seem such an outlandish idea? We require a certain chronological maturity for driving a car, for buying a drink, for registering for the draft, and for voting. Sexual activity is as important as all of them and more vital than some of them. In view of all the factors in the situation, it is very hard to find any way of twisting things around to say that the ethics of teen-age relationships make sexual activity at an early age justified.

"Everyone says for us to stay out of trouble and don't mess around, but there is really almost nothing else to do."

I understand, and I know this is your most difficult problem. You must pay adult prices at the movies, and then the picture is loaded with bedroom scenes. You may bowl a few games, or skate, but these activities take money, too, and you don't feel athletic on every date. I know you are not welcome in a lot of places. They don't want you sitting around their restaurants or standing around on their parking lots. The adults who keep telling you to stay out of trouble have no time to set up recreational activities for you or to find good places in which you can spend your free time. They are probably too busy

YOU AND THE NO-NO'S

making the money for you to spend. It is a vicious circle, and you wind up sitting in the dark in a parked car, or back at the movies again, watching somebody on the screen make love.

In general I would say that the more single-dating you do, the more sex problems you have. Getting involved in group activities seems to lessen the tensions. Also, girls tell me this is safer for their reputations. When everyone is together, it is harder for rumors to start, and girls find that their dates are much less likely to try things when there is no doubt about the girl's standards.

"It doesn't always work out that way. Some boys are very nice when you have them alone, but in front of a crowd they act up and show off."

That figures, I suppose, with certain types. It is possible, too, that if you happen to be with a fast crowd, the pressure on the individual to do what the others are doing would be great.

"That's right. If you are with a crowd, and everyone starts making out, it is very hard to handle it. But if you are on a single date, and the fellow wants to start something, you can usually talk it over."

It sounds as though times have changed, and we must take another look at the idea that crowd-dating is safer. I suppose, from what you say, that a couple who went in for heavy petting would do it anyway, in spite of the crowd.

It sounds as though you are going to need to work this problem out together, by talking it over and finding the best solution for you in view of what the rest of the crowd will be doing. It seems logical to say that maybe you had better pick your crowd pretty carefully. If those in the In Group are going to devote their evenings to sex, maybe you will want to conclude that the price of admission to that crowd is too steep.

Perhaps, then, we had better examine another old standby: Going steady creates more sex problems than going with a lot of people.

"That is still true, and I wanted to ask about it. My girl and I have been going together for a year, and I really care for her. I don't want to do anything to hurt her. But when we are together, we just want each other. Neither of us wants to go with anyone else. We tried it, and we don't have any fun."

You had better find a mutual hobby. I mean it. Crossword or jigsaw puzzles. Building model airplanes. Making sailing ships inside of bottles. Jogging. Catching butterflies. Laughter: laughter is very good for sexual tension. Kid each other out of it. Be sensitive to the other's mood, and try to head in the other direction when you see trouble coming. If you can, find a crowd that doesn't go in for the sort of thing that gives you a problem. Maybe you can find a club made up of middle-aged joggers or something.

"Sometimes when you listen to discussions, you get the feeling people still think sex is dirty."

Well, let's take care of that right now. The human body is beautiful, and the right kind of sex is beautiful, too.

YOU AND THE NO-NO'S

A lot of the problems that arise in marriage come from the opposite idea. When I counsel people who are about to be married, I always tell them—even though sometimes they are shocked—that as long as the two people keep their bodies clean, there is nothing they can do that is wrong or dirty. This feeling that sex is dirty stems, not from the right kind of sex, but from the wrong kind.

You know, a knife is not intrinsically evil. It is the use you make of it that determines whether it is evil or not. You can use a knife to cut bread, or you can use it to stab someone.

It is the same way with sex. It can be useful and beautiful, or it can be a terrible thing, depending on the way it is used. Sex, in itself, is no more sinful than a table knife. Sin comes from using sex—or the knife—in an evil way. The evil side of sex comes, as we have said, from approaching it with the idea, "What's in it for me?"

When you have a relationship with another human being, you are not tinkering with an object. You are not playing with a toy. This is another *person*. This is a collection of real feelings.

Remember the old story about how God made the oyster? He put all the sensitive organism on the inside, protected by a hard, bony shell. It is very difficult to hurt an oyster, and an oyster never learns anything. But when God made people, the story goes, he did just the opposite. He put the hard, bony substance on the inside and the delicate, tender flesh on the outside. So people feel things. They suffer, and they can be hurt. And they can learn and be wise.

The question you must ask yourself is, "What am I

doing to this other human being?" If you are really being loving, if you are truly *aware* of the other as a sensitive, perceptive individual, you will make any sacrifice to spare this loved one the slightest pain or mental anguish.

Selfish people are never aware of another person. They do not even hear another's voice. Life, for them, is a long monologue. Unselfishness is genuinely caring about another's well-being, another's happiness, another's reputation. It is total awareness of another's primary needs. This kind of love—this kind of sex—is beautiful.

"I don't really want to go against my inner standards, but when I try to explain, and people argue with me, I can't think of any reason not to do what they say. All I can tell them is, something inside me won't let me. And the kids say, 'You're just immature, you'll change.' And I keep wondering, will I?"

Now you know how a conscientious objector feels. That's what you are, you know. In the sexual revolution you are a conscientious objector. I know it takes courage.

It has been said that religion is not a way of looking at certain things; it is, rather, a certain way of looking at everything. Now it is very hard to keep in mind your personal ethics, your personal point of view, if you are going to think about it in terms of one small part of your life—in this case, in regard to your social life and your desire to have friends. But when you apply your personal point of view to your *whole life*, the picture comes into focus much better. Then you are looking at what you want for yourself, in the long-range view. You are trying to find the you-ness of you. You are looking for the

YOU AND THE NO-NO'S

dimensions of your own unique identity as a child of God. Or, if you prefer to keep the discussion nonreligious, you are seeking to understand your individual nature as a member of that species which has been called "the climax of creation." You are seeking the best way to use your abilities, which are nowhere exactly duplicated.

Now the decisions you make on a day-to-day basis must be related to this long-range view of your life. It is very hard to think of intelligent reasons for the choices you make if you are surrounded by people who are living as though there were not going to be any tomorrow. This is exactly what that inner code of yours is saying: There is a tomorrow, and it is very important to me. I want to live today in a way that will enhance and not jeopardize my tomorrow.

This is true self-respect. It is the highest kind of self-love. It includes a genuine and really humble reverence for the awesome mystery of individual identity. There is nothing egotistical about it. It relates also to the kind of love you can give to another person. If you are clear about yourself, the love you give another is freely given. It does not grow out of dissatisfaction with yourself, some need you want the other person to supply. It is, put another way, true maturity.

"Then what you are saying is, you can't find out what to do by turning to the Bible and looking something up. You have to more or less play everything by ear."

Yes, not because the Bible doesn't have the answers—it does—but in this day people want first to find the answer for themselves. As someone said earlier, her mother talks about God's law, and the magazines talk about the death of God. So what we must find is a lightweight, portable, and up-to-date code of morals that will wear well and not become obsolete, can be easily adapted to our changing needs, and will guarantee good results no matter how far away from home we get.

This personal morality is a private luxury. Sometimes it costs us a great deal. Like any precious possession, it occasionally arouses envy in others. We may find people trying to take it away from us. We see the great need to take good care of this personal treasure, for the sake of others as well as for our own sake. It is often the only way we can help people we are concerned about. It is one of those rare gifts you can share with others and never find diminishing.

Of the boys it demands an ever-growing manhood. Of the girls it demands an early willingness to take on one of the roles women have historically assumed—that of setting the moral tone of society. Or to use the words of a young man I know, "The day a girl learns to say 'no' is the day she becomes a real girl."

This new morality is so much purer than the old. Instead of being based on fear of all those great, booming No-No's, it concerns itself with responsible living—with responsible sexuality—in the interests of a better life for ourselves, and for those we love, and for everyone.

Bibliography

I. SELECTED REFERENCES ON ASPECTS OF SEX EDUCATION
   A. Guides for parents and teachers
      Bibby, Cyril. *Sex Education: A Guide for Parents, Teachers, and Youth Leaders.* New York: Emerson Books, 1944.

      Facts Aren't Enough. (Pamphlet) American Medical Association, 535 N. Dearborn Street, Chicago 10, Ill.

      Glover, Leland E. *How to Help Your Teen-Ager Grow Up.* New York: P. F. Collier, 1962.

      Hymes, James L., Jr. *How to Tell Your Child About Sex.* (Pamphlet) Public Affairs Committee, 22 East 38th Street, New York, N. Y. 10016.

      Is There a Morals Revolt Among Youth? (Pamphlet) American Social Health Association, 1790 Broadway, New York, N. Y. 10019.

      Know Your Daughter. (Pamphlet) American Social Health Association.

      Know Your Son. (Pamphlet) American Social Health Association.

Lerrigo, Marion O. and Helen Southard. *Sex Facts and Attitudes*. New York: E. P. Dutton, 1956.

Loeb, Martin S. *Sex Role and Identity in Adolescence*. (Pamphlet) American Social Health Association.

Parents' Guide to the Facts of Life. (Pamphlet) Child Study Association of America, 9 East 89th Street, New York, N. Y. 10028.

Parents' Privilege. (Pamphlet) American Medical Association.

Terry, Luther L. *VD's Alarming Comeback*. Reprinted from *Look*, December 4, 1962. Copies may be obtained from the Communicable Disease Center of the Public Health Service, 1600 Clifton Road, N. E., Atlanta, Ga.

What to Tell Your Children About Sex. (Pamphlet) Child Study Association of America.

When Children Ask About Sex. (Pamphlet) Child Study Association of America.

B. To be read to little children

Buck, Pearl. *Johnny Jack and His Beginnings*. New York: The John Day Co., 1954.

Faegre, Marion L. *Your Own Story*. Minneapolis: University of Minnesota Press, 1943.

Facts of Life for Children. (Pamphlet) Child Study Association of America.

Gruenberg, Sidonie M. *The Wonderful Story of How You Were Born*. Garden City, N. Y.: Doubleday & Co., 1952.

de Schweinitz, Karl. *Growing Up*. New York: The Macmillan Co., 1953.

A Story About You. (Pamphlet) American Medical Association.

BIBLIOGRAPHY: BOOKS AND FILMS ABOUT SEX

C. Older children and young adolescents

Beck, Lester F. *Human Growth.* New York: Harcourt, Brace & World, 1949.

Boys Want to Know. (Pamphlet) American Social Health Association.

Corner, George W. *Attaining Manhood.* New York: Harper & Row, 1952.

———. *Attaining Womanhood.* New York: Harper & Row, 1952.

Dating Days. (Pamphlet) American Social Health Association.

Force, Elizabeth S. *Your Family Today and Tomorrow.* New York: Harcourt, Brace & World, 1955.

Gruenberg, Benjamin C. and Sidonie. *The Wonderful Story of You.* Garden City, N. Y.: Doubleday & Co., 1960.

Landis, Paul H. *Coming of Age: Problems of Teen-Agers.* (Pamphlet) Public Affairs Pamphlets, 22 East 38th Street, New York, N. Y. 10016.

Let's Tell the Whole Story About Sex. (Pamphlet) American Social Health Association.

Levine, Milton and Jean Seligmann. *The Wonder of Life.* New York: Golden Press, 1952.

Meugarten, Bernice L. *Becoming Men and Women.* Science Research Associates, Inc., 259 East Erie Street, Chicago 11, Ill.

D. Older adolescents and young adults

Duvall, Evelyn Millis, *Love and the Facts of Life.* New York: Association Press, 1963.

——— and Reuben Hill. *When You Marry.* New York: Association Press, 1962.

Everyone Should Know. (Pamphlet) American Social Health Association.

Finding Yourself. (Pamphlet) American Medical Association.

Gottlieb, Bernard S. and Sophie B. *What You Should Know About Marriage.* Indianapolis: Bobbs-Merrill, 1962.

Landis, Judson T. and Mary G. *Building a Successful Marriage.* 4th ed. Englewood Cliffs, N. J.: Prentice-Hall, 1963.

Learning About Love. (Pamphlet) American Medical Association.

Strictly for Teen-Agers. Department of Health, Education, and Welfare, Public Health Service, PHSP No. 913, U. S. Government Printing Office, Washington, D. C. 20401.

II. FILMS FOR USE IN SEX EDUCATION (16 MM.)

A. The facts of sex

Boy to Man. Churchill Films, 662 N. Robertson Blvd., Los Angeles, Calif. 90069.

From Generation to Generation. McGraw-Hill Book Co., 330 West 42nd Street, New York, N. Y. 10036.

Girl to Woman. Churchill Films.

Human and Animal Beginnings. E. C. Brown Trust, 3170 S. W. 87th Avenue, Portland Oregon 97225.

Human Growth. E. C. Brown Trust.

Human Reproduction. McGraw-Hill Book Co.

B. Dating, love, and sex relations

The Game. McGraw-Hill Book Co.

The Merry-Go-Round. McGraw-Hill Book Co.

Worth Waiting For. Brigham Young University, Provo, Utah.

C. The problems of illegitimacy

Phoebe. McGraw-Hill Book Co.

A Statistic Named Ann. WJZ-TV (Westinghouse Broadcasting), Television Hill, Baltimore, Md. 21211.

D. Family relationships

Parents are People, Too. McGraw-Hill Book Co.

Parent to Child About Sex. Wayne State University, Detroit, Mich.

The Teens. McGraw-Hill Book Co.

E. Preparation for marriage

Beyond Conception. Popular Dynamics, 13201 Ninth, N. W., Seattle, Wash. 98177.

Children by Choice. Planned Parenthood-World Population, 515 Madison Avenue, New York, N. Y. 10022.

Early Marriage. E. C. Brown Trust.

Fair Chance. Parthenon Pictures, 2625 Temple Street, Los Angeles, Calif. 90026.

Introduction to Birth Control Methods. Planned Parenthood-World Population.

It Takes All Kinds. McGraw-Hill Book Co.,

This Charming Couple. McGraw-Hill Book Co.

Walt Disney's *Family Planning.* Buena Vista Productions, 800 Sonora Avenue, Glendale, Calif. 91201.

Who's Boss? McGraw-Hill Book Co.

The addresses given with the above list of films indicate the source from which the films may be purchased. Many of them can, however, be rented from Yeshiva University Film Library, 526 West 187th Street, New York, N. Y. 10033.

III. SELECTED FICTION ON SEXUAL PROBLEMS

Sometimes young people can learn much from becoming emotionally involved in a work of fiction and then discussing the characters' problems. The following titles are works of fiction in which young people come face to face with sexual problems (except the last one, which is the autobiography of an unwed mother).

Baker, Laura	*Go Away, Ruthie*
Bawden, Nina	*Tortoise by Candlelight*
Craig, Margaret	*It Could Happen to Anyone*
Eyerly, Jeannette	*A Girl Like Me*
Felsen, Henry Gregor	*Two and the Town*
Head, Ann	*Mr. and Mrs. Bo Jo Jones*
McCullers, Carson	*The Heart Is a Lonely Hunter*
McCullers, Carson	*Member of the Wedding*
Parks, Gordon	*The Learning Tree*
Perrin, Ursula	*Ghosts*
Price, Reynolds	*A Long and Happy Life*
Salinger, J. D.	*The Catcher in the Rye*
Sherburne, Zoa	*Too Bad About the Haines Girl*
Smith, Betty	*Joy in the Morning*
Smith, Betty	*A Tree Grows in Brooklyn*
Stolz, Mary	*A Love or a Season*
Stolz, Mary	*Second Nature*
Wouk, Herman	*Marjorie Morningstar*
Thompson, Jean	*The House of Tomorrow*

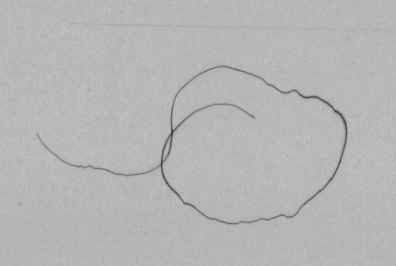